How To Improve Your Sex Life

Matt ～ Ville

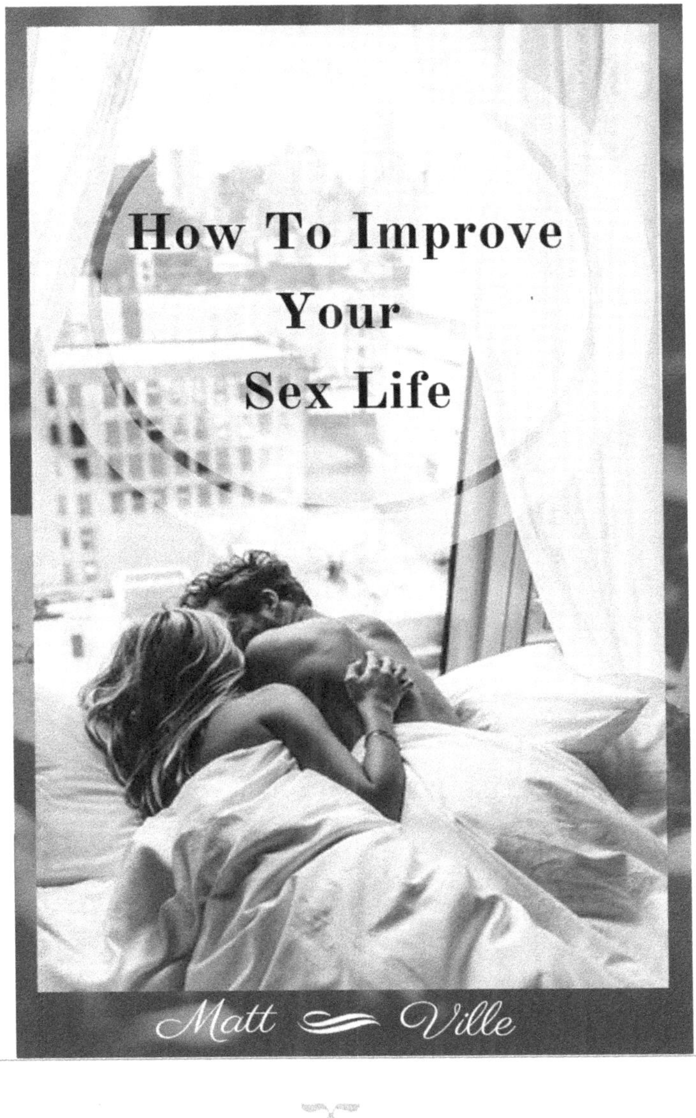

HOW TO IMPROVE YOUR SEX LIFE

By

MattVille'

Copyright

INTRODUCTION

The secret to a good sex life, and to a good life in general, is quite simply this: learn to communicate effectively. No trick, position, sex toy or "new" experience will make sex better if we haven't learned the most fundamental and most powerful skill any person could have namely to listen and to respond effectively. This skill is particularly difficult between the two sexes because men use different parts of their brain to listen and respond than women do. That being said, the fact that we use different parts of our brains to communicate works out perfectly in nature and therefore becomes critical in a good sex life.

The ultimate expression

In kindergarten we are taught that we listen with our ears. This isn't so - our ears receive sound waves, but it is our brains that do the listening. Moreover, if we take body language into account, we receive signals with our eyes as well. When it comes to sex, not only do we see body language, we also feel signals, hear signals, smell signals and taste signals. Sex is the ultimate form of communication. The entire body tells a story that combines smells, and tastes and feelings and sounds into the pinnacle of pleasure.

The thing with sex though is that, because our entire body speaks, it reflects our mind completely. We cannot separate our minds from our bodies, especially when we are giving ourselves so completely. This is precisely where the catch comes in - all our fears, inhibitions and uncertainties are reflected along with our hopes and expectations. This is the key to understanding sex: fear holds us back, freedom allows us greater experiences. Therefore, we must be free to communicate in order to have better sex!

To listen and respond

We may all use the same words, and roughly construct sentences in the same way, but each and every human being has a language of their own. As babies we responded to our mother's touch, as children we learned the meaning of words through our personal experiences. As teenagers we developed a deeper value to these words and as adults we use them to be productive. Our understanding of language is subject to so many variations in our experiences that each one of us has a unique language. How we get along is a miracle - mostly our need to survive overrides the potential conflicts of the misunderstandings we regularly have.

I grew up in the 80's and 90's when "Women's Lib" was at a peak - as a boy I was taught that men must listen to women, but because no man in my previous generation knew precisely what that entails, I developed a low self esteem when it came to girls. I felt inadequate when it came to understanding them and listening to them because every effort I made somehow failed to make an impression. It was only when I met a girl who didn't expect me to know everything beforehand that I was able to start learning.

After many years of good relationships and many intimate experiences, I discovered a simple way to learn a woman's language: ask. When you are doing something new with your hands, listen to her breathing, feel the response of her body, listen to the sounds she is making - when they all tell you that it is good, then chances are that it is good. However, girls sometimes make the same noises during sex that they make when digging out dish washing liquid under the sink, and that is when us men get really confused. Instead of trying to guess whether that was a "oh my gosh do it again" groan or a "that's not it!" groan, simply ask whether what you are doing works for her. If it does, keep going. If it doesn't, ask her to move your hand, or simply try something new. Soon you will learn what noises and body movements equate to a good time, and which ones equate to discomfort.

Being able to ask shows a great deal of maturity and confidence - these are two highly sought after characteristics that will add to the entire sex experience. Using this method of exploration I was able to learn very quickly what a particular girl likes or dislikes and by doing what works I had some of the best experiences one could ask for.

The risk of exposing oneself

The idea of sex as the ultimate form of communication is as much a blessing as it can be a curse. Most people know this instinctively, and when it comes to sex they try to manage the risk of exposing themselves so blatantly by withholding on some areas and overemphasizing others. Sex simply isn't at its utmost best if you can't give or receive everything, completely. So learning the secret language she uses to reveal herself will take time. Don't expect amazing sex in one night stands - good sex sometimes happens, but if the sex was good for that single instance, imagine what it would be if you actually knew her!

The reluctance we have in opening ourselves up so completely can be a very healthy thing. It allows us to limit our emotional involvement and gives us time to ensure that we have selected a good mate. This is why sex in longer term relationships get better (presuming that the partners work on it). In some cases however childhood experiences, social norms or some belief may inhibit us sexually in unhealthy ways. As the man in the relationship this is your task: to navigate through these fears and inhibitions so that you can release the passion in your partner.

This is precisely where the story comes together- the better we know someone, the better the sex. In fact, the old Hebrew word for sex used in the Bible means "to know". Whether you believe in the Bible or not is irrelevant, the fact is that an ancient culture understood that sex is equal to knowledge. Truly knowing her is the key to unlocking the passion in your relationship.

WHAT IS SEX COACHING?

Deciding to contact another person, who you don't know, in order to discuss your sexual concerns can be rather daunting. I would like you to be able to understand what sex coaching is, what it can do for you, how it works and what your contribution to the process is, so that you can then be in the best position to choose the most appropriate course of action to resolve your sexual difficulties.

Most sex advice in popular media relies on giving you tips and tricks to impress and tantalize your lover. If you are in a sexual relationship that is not working, merely doing something different is unlikely to resolve your concerns and it could exacerbate them. I do understand that it sounds appealing to be able to save your sex life by finding new things to do. A quick fix sounds good. It takes minimal effort and promises maximum gains. The actual physical aspect of sexual stimulation is only one part of desire and arousal. Sometimes, when you reduce people to a series of new and potentially undiscovered body parts, sexual connection breaks down even further. You may find new ways to arouse them sexually, but that does not mean that sexual fulfilment is any closer for either of you.

What many people fail to realise is that sexual arousal is both physical and mental. Probably many of us have experienced being with a partner who is technically proficient but who seems cold and disconnected from us. Most people like to feel that their partner is emotionally 'there' with them, not just with another body, who could belong to anyone. This counts for both casual and longer-term relationships. There is a vast difference between being sexually competent and deeply pleasuring your partner. Your mind and emotions play a key role in how you receive and what you feel about physical pleasure. If your partner seems emotionally distant but physically experienced, many people then start to worry about their own 'performance' and physical appearance. The sex-self-spirit connection takes into account the thoughts, feelings, emotions and beliefs that you have that are part of all your sexual experiences.

Of course, when things start to improve, there is nothing wrong with looking for innovative sexual behaviours to experiment with. As long as you are not trying to fix something merely by touching someone on a new part of their body or with a different sort of pressure, sexual exploration can bring you closer together. Remember though that everyone responds differently and not all the 'tricks' you learn are going to work with everybody. Part of the fun is finding out which ones do.

On a very basic level, sex coaching - like all forms of coaching - is basically a conversation. It just happens to focus upon sexual matters. We talk about your sexual behaviours, the way you feel about yourself as a sexual person and the things you are afraid of. Coaching conversations are distinctive in many ways form the type of discussion you would normally have. We work with feelings, thoughts, beliefs and values that are under the surface; facets that are part of you and that partially determine how you think and act but that are largely unquestioned and often retain their power way beyond the time when they may originally have been useful.

Having a fulfilling sex life builds self-confidence, self-esteem and personal empowerment. Sadly, many people expect sex to always work 'naturally' and 'magically'. It doesn't. Not always. Almost everyone will experience some kind of sexual concern at one point; whether it be low arousal, lack of sexual desire, inability to orgasm, being too quick to orgasm, sexual pain and discomfort, worries about ageing, inhibition due to concerns about body image. People would often rather live in denial rather than face up to the fact that they are not having the sex that they would like to have. Sexual problems are not disasters. They are normal and natural and completely open to resolution.

When I coach I help people to work out what their specific Sex Goals are; what do you really want? What are the underlying issues? Do you lack the knowledge, experience or courage to communicate? Do you wish your partner connected with you more emotionally? Or helped you feel more wanted, valued, desirable? Equally as important is acknowledging the current state of your sex life. What is missing? What precisely is not working? Often, the deeper issues are not the ones that you thought they were.

Personal empowerment is a fundamental goal of all good coaching. The greatest mark of success is when you finish your coaching sessions and leave, happy that your present circumstances have changed for the better - you have reached, maybe even surpassed, your Sex Goals - and knowing that you can trust yourself to deal with whatever happens in the future.

Sex coaching helps you expand your choices

One of the distinctive aspects of coaching is that the coach does not have the answers. YOU have the answers. Most of the time we do things and believe things without really questioning our reasons. We get into habits of thought and action that prevent us from looking for alternatives. Sex coaching helps you recognise that there are different choices that you can make, which will enable you to enjoy better sex and experience more of your sexual potential.

Usually you don't get a chance to explore your own deeper feelings because people like to 'fix' other people. Your friends and family jump in with their advice and their suggestions before you have had the chance to deeply examine the choices that you want to make. This is why coaching is such a powerful form of personal growth. It helps you know that you can resolve your own problems. Many people find that, once they have created a fulfilling sex life, there are other aspects of their life that they wish to change. Many people feel powerless because they don't take the chance with themselves to see and find out what they are capable of. When you refuse to settle for a second-rate sex life, you are probably no longer - for example - willing to work in a job that you hate for the rest of your life. Recognise this: you are quite capable of being brave, finding creative alternatives and making change happen.

Awareness and Responsibility

This might not sound very sexy but becoming more aware and embracing a sense of personal responsibility are two of the most valuable and liberating things that you can do. The power of both of these lies in the fact that they give you control and increase your belief in your ability to influence and change any situation. Trying to deal with sexual problems can easily deteriorate into a heated and angry exchange of blame, denial, justification and criticism.

Most of us would rather believe that we are faultless and the problem lies with some inadequacy or insensitivity within the other person. How is this presumption ever going to lead to an improvement in your sexual relationship? Simple, it just is not going to. Any problem that two people have with any kind of relationship between them is something that both have created. The great thing is that it only takes one of you to commit to change to make change happen.

What do you really pay for when you choose to work with a sex coach?

You have the chance to talk to someone about very profound aspects of your life without having to worry that they are going to jump in and offer inappropriate advice and try and steer you to reach the same decision that they would make.

You have permission to talk about anything that is troubling you and need not be concerned about being judged, mocked or condemned for anything you want to do, say or feel.

You do not have to impress me. Sex coaching is one of the few times when you can talk about sex without fear of having to match up to any spurious standard or norm of behaviour or desire.
You get the chance to discover that you are as attractive and desirable as you think that you are. Sexual attraction is often idiosyncratic and unpredictable because sexuality is about more than appearance. It's about energy and confidence and communication.

Get in touch to arrange an initial conversation about sex coaching. You will get to know me a bit better and decide for yourself whether you are ready to explore and discover how great you are and how wondrous and magnificent your sex life can be.

WHAT IS A NORMAL SEX LIFE?

This survey is not the truth of sexual activity in Britain but it is a useful way in to talk about common questions that I get asked.

SEXUAL EXPERIENCE - how many sexual partners have you had?

The average person has had 9 sexual partners, although averages are pretty meaningless figures in themselves. More interesting is the fact that only 20% of the population have had more than 10 sexual partners. People often tell me that their lack of experience makes them feel sexually unadventurous and this impinges upon their confidence. There seems to be an assumption that the more partners you have, the better lover you are or the more 'sexual' you are as a person. Neither of these is true and most people imagine that other people have way more partners than they actually do. Quality counts, not quantity. I don't think it is difficult to build up a pretty large number of partners. Much more tricky to actually focus on having a mutually enjoyable sexual encounter.

SEXUAL CONFIDENCE - how would you rate your sexual performance?

One of the things that undermines people's belief in the inheherent 'rightness' of their own sexuality is assuming that other people are more skilled and better lovers than we are . 24% rate their sexual performance as very good . This means that three-quarters of us think that we are, at best good and at worst, very poor in bed. Many people are anxious about sex, forgetting that the identity of our partner impacts upon sexual performance. Performance is really all about confidence and having a partner who supports your belief in your desirability makes you a good lover with that person. Sex shouldn't be a performance. If it is, your beliefs about sex could benefit from some self-reflection and examination. Focusing on your own performance makes you want to please your partner in order to uphold your own self-esteem rather than wanting to give pleasure for the sake of it.

SEXUAL SATISFACTION - are you currently satisfied with your sex life?

76% said yes, 24% said no. A quarter of people cannot find a way to create the kind of sexual connections and experiences that they would like to be having. This result is unusual as typically most surveys report over 50% dissatisfaction rates. Those aged 65 and over were more satisfied than those aged 16-24. People in long-term relationships/marriage are more satisfied than single people, although single people report having sex more often. Again, frequency is no guarantee of good sex. Nor is youth and beauty. Of course, we don't know what satisfied means to the people who answered the questions. No sex can be satisfactory for some people. In fact , 36% of 16-24 year olds believe that it is possible to have a happy relationship/marriage without sex.

SEXUAL FREQUENCY - how often do you have sex?

I think this is THE most common worry that people have. Am I having sex often enough? Is my level of desire normal? 25% do not have any sex in an average month . Not everybody is having a lot of sex and it is likely that many of those are perfectly happy with their situation. Another 25% have sex between 6-10 times a month. Most people do not, except maybe at the beginning of a relationship, have vast amounts of sex all the time. A lot of people believe that everyone has more sex than they do. And they worry about this. Frequency needs to be looked at in relation to satisfaction before people start getting concerned about how much or how little they have sex. If you're happy and your partner is satisfied, then you're lucky - regardless of how little or often you are actually having sex.

SEXUAL DESIRE - how do you rate your sex drive?

Levels of desire is another area that people get hung up about. People worry, should I want to have sex more than I actually do? In the survey 32% rate their sex drive as average , 24% describe their libido as low or very low. Most people do not see themselves as possessing a high sex drive. Only 1 in 5 rate their sex drive as very high. Desire ebbs and flows and this is normal and to be expected.

Sexual honesty and deep conversation about sex with a range of people is not something that many of us are lucky enough to experience. We rely on our assumptions, insecurities and fears to 'imagine' that other people's sexual experiences are more frequent, enjoyable and adventurous than our own. Whilst surveys give us averages and the ordinary, they can also reveal that sexuality is diverse and normality is difficult - and rather pointless - to define.

WHO WANTS TO BE NORMAL?

What makes us so afraid to stand up and stand out when it comes to our sexuality? Most people play safe and so do not enable their sexual potential to be explored and attained. The crucial question to ask yourself is:

If I am NOT sexually normal, what does it mean?

Each of us will have our own reasons as to what it means if we feel that our sexual desires, tastes and experiences are not the same as most other people's. We are free to choose what our sexuality means and not to be dictated to by cultural standards of acceptability. One size does not fit all when it comes to the magnificent variety of preferences, needs, desires, beliefs and opinions that we hold.

It doesn't mean that we all worry that we are too sexually outrageous. Some may feel that if they don't want sex 'enough' then they are just not very sexual people, which can soon become a belief that one is not desirable and so does not deserve anything else. We forget that sexuality changes over years and from day to day and so defining ones sexuality is not a fixed and final process.

As well as reassuring people that 'normal' sexuality is impossible to define, I also discuss the what it means to them to be normal. Why do they seem to want their sexuality to be sanctioned by its apparent ordinariness? This gets to the root of fears about sex and what sex represents. Addressing such concerns contributes to a big increase in people's confidence, authenticity and self-acceptance.

SAFER SEX MENU

Safer sex can be fun and you won't have to worry as much. The best advice is to use safer sex supplies until you and your lover are in a monogamous relationship.

- Saucy phone-sex or sex talk
- A luscious body massage
- Naughty videos & audios
- Scrumptious body licking
- A spicy striptease
- Savory kissing
- Mouth watering mutual masturbation
- Tasty cleavage fornication
- Juicy oral delights with a condom or rubber dam
- Steamy sex with vibrators and other adult toys (Not shared)
- Delicious penetration with an FDA approved condom

- Sugary caresses
- Syrupy love bites served gently
- Sweet body pressing
- Warm blows of breath

- Creamy cuddles

Condom Talk

If your lover gives you a hard time about wearing a condom, here are some good responses and excellent reasons why you need to use one.

- Him: I don't think condoms are romantic.
- Her: Just let me show you how romantic condoms can be.
- Him: You don't trust me, do you?
- Her: It's not a matter of trust; it's a matter of health.
- Him: I don't like to use condoms.
- Her: I don't have sex without them.
- Him: I haven't had sex with anyone in years so I know I'm clean.

- Her: Thanks for being so honest, but let's use one anyway.
- Him: I can't feel anything when I wear a condom.
- Her: Let me provide you with some extra stimulation.
- Him: I know I'll lose my erection by the time I get it on.
- Her: Here, let me put it on for you with my mouth.
- Him: I'm only going to use a condom this once.
- Her: Once is all it takes.
- Him: Sorry, I don't have one.
- Her: That's ok. I do.
- Him: How come you have condoms on you? Did you plan to have sex with me?
- Her: I made sure I had some because I really care about you.
- Him: Forget it. I'm not going to use a condom.
- Her: Fine. Then let's not have sex until we can work out our differences.

Who needs it and why use it?

Superstar athletes, actors, rock stars, politicians, even entrepreneurs have groupies that will do just about anything to have sex with them, but can they be trusted? Will they lie about the act being consensual? Could they threaten to sue or worse still, make an accusation about sexual assault? You bet they can! So how can these people who are regularly out of town and away from home, which can lead to loneliness and result in temptation, protect themselves? Condoms can protect from the Std's and unwanted pregnancy. Another form of protection is to have a signed sexual consent form before having any sex as I described on TV's Celebrity Justice, CNN , ABC , Fox News and Good Morning America

If you think that a sexual consent form is only for the rich and famous, think again. Even if you have no assets, you need to protect yourself from false accusations because you can lose everything including your personal property, freedom and reputation. There are many other benefits to signing a sexual consent form, including the fact that you literally open up a form of intimate communication prior to rushing into sex. And, ladies the sexual consent form can protect you from being taken advantage of sexually because there is an -out clause- that stipulates that if you say the words -Code Red,- your partner must stop immediately. I chose this phrase because the words -No- and -Stop- have been used all too frivolously in our society and unfortunately, they are not always taken seriously. By using the sexual consent form with an FDA approved condom, you could protect yourself legally and sexually.

Benefits of a Sexual Consent Form

- I created it so that there will be no confusion or miscommunication as far as sexual consent is concerned.
- It protects men from conniving women who may bring false charges of sexual misconduct for financial gain.
- Even men who have no assets need to protect themselves from false accusations because they can lose everything that is dearest to them. Property, freedom and their reputation.
- This form is actually a way for the man to ask for permission to have sex with the woman.
- Women should NOT sign it if they do not trust the man are not ready for intimacy.
- It can be a form of foreplay before you get to the bedroom since you get to talk about sex before rushing into it. Great communication.
- The woman can select which sexual activities she wants to indulge in.
- -No- & -Stop- has been used frivolously, playfully and teasingly & is not taken seriously anymore. The phrase Code Red will not be mistaken for anything other than -high alert- hands off, you've gone too far. A similar 'Out Clause' is used in consensual bondage.
- Code Red is an alert that means stop because I am having physical or emotional problems. He must stop instantly.
- Any contract is contestable, even a prenuptial or Will. But if I were accused, I would rather go to court with it than without it. It would

be admissible and relevant as evidence of consent if signed by the alleged victim.

· It's a great way to keep tabs on how many sex partners you've had.

· This is not a rape tool. On the contrary, I believe that it will prevent rape. A rapist is less likely to use a sexual consent form.

· As for the argument that a woman can be forced into signing it, I contend that a handwriting expert could probably identify a forced signature.

· There is never a guarantee that someone will NOT take advantage of you sexually, emotionally or physically. The best line of defence is always to be cautious and listen to your gut instincts. Never do anything that you do not want to do!

Is Oral Sex really Sex?

It is ridiculous to view oral sex as -not sex.- It's just as intimate as sexual intercourse, so why would you engage in oral sex with someone you wouldn't want to have intercourse with? Well, I'll tell you why. It all started in 1998 when then President Bill Clinton stated publicly, -I did not have sexual relations with that woman- even though he had repeatedly received oral sex from his intern, Monica Lewinsky. Now there is the growing problem of defining what sex really is. In the minds of many teenagers, oral sex isn't really sex. They seem to think they can stay virgins by engaging in oral sex because their hymen isn't broken. That's like saying, you can have anal sex and remain a virgin. Technically, it's true, but theoretically and emotionally it's not. Some guys also think they aren't cheating when they have oral sex with another woman because they can't get her pregnant. Giving and receiving oral sex is one of the most intimate and erotic acts that can be exchanged within a loving adult relationship and yes, it is sex!
Oral sex isn't a safe sex activity

Although oral sex is safer than vaginal and anal sex, it is still possible to contract Std's. The bottom line is that oral sex should be avoided if the giver has any sores or bleeding gums in the mouth. Even if he or she has just brushed or flossed their teeth, it can cause microscopic scratches in the lining of the mouth that makes one vulnerable to infection. Because of this, doctors advise the use of condoms for fellatio (flavored condoms are best) and the use of female condoms, dental dams or kitchen plastic wrap) for cunnilingus.

Better to be safe than sorry

Many people are unclear on the risks associated with oral sex. Unprotected oral sex carries a lesser risk for the transmission of sexually transmitted diseases (Std's) than unprotected intercourse or anal penetration, but there's still a risk for both the giver and the receiver of oral sex. First let's look at how to avoid these contagious Std's by practicing safer sex.

Safer Sex Supplies

If you love yourself, you must protect yourself. Ladies, there's no reason why you can't enjoy the eroticism of oral sex and practice safer sex at the same time. Even if you're in a monogamous relationship, you'll want to have some of the safer sex supplies around to help you add more pleasure, persity and spontaneity to your oral sex adventures.

Female Condoms

Reality Condoms are the most well known, but they recently changed their name to FC Female Condoms. Femidom is another brand of female condoms. Most female condoms work the same way. They're made of polyurethane (stronger than latex), are hypo-allergenic, heat conductive, and odorless. They are a soft, loose-fitting sheath specifically designed to protect women from pregnancy and Std's by lining the inside of her vagina. Read the instructions before inserting it because if you don't insert it correctly, it's like not using protection at all. The female condom has to go deep inside the vagina and over the cervix.

Dental Dams

Aptly named because they are used by dentists to isolate a tooth. Dental dams come in various sizes and flavors. Made of ultra think latex, these square shaped barriers allow good sensations for oral sex. Sheer Glyde Dams are FDA approved for protection against Std's for cunnilingus and rimming. The best way to use a dam is for the giver to mark the -mouth-side of the dam with a marker so that they knows which side to lick, then apply a couple of drops of lubricant on the other side, press the dam against her vulva with two hands and enjoy.

Latex Gloves and Finger Cots

Good oral sex involves the hands as well as the mouth. There's nothing more exciting than orally pleasing a woman's clitoris and fingering her vagina or anus simultaneously. By using latex gloves and or finger cots (think of them as mini condoms for your fingers) you can increase erotic sensations and protect the receiver from jagged fingernails, cuts, germs or viral Std's such as herpes, which can be spread by skin-to-skin contact.

Lubricants

We all know, -wetter is better.- But, which lube is best? It can be very confusing because there are so many to choose from including, odorless, tasteless, water soluble lubricants with a lightconsistency and without Nonoxynol-9 spermicide. Here are some favorites: Wet Light, Astroglide, ForePlay Personal Gel, Aqua Lube, Sensua Organics and Probe Silky Light.

What Stds can I get from Oral Sex?

The following list of Std's is the most contagious and common when it comes to performing and receiving oral sex on a person. While no one knows exactly what the degree of risk is, to ensure safeties make sure that no cuts or lesions are present in the mouth or on the genitals.

Protect yourself and your partner by using a barrier to avoid the contact of bodily fluids that may result in catching a sexually transmitted disease.

Herpes is a virus that causes sporadic flare-ups of painful blisters, usually around the mouth and or genitals. Herpes can hop from mouth to mouth and from mouth to genitals through the mucous membranes and skin. It can be spread by hand to vagina or hand to anus contact. Since Herpes is such a common virus, you can get a prescription drug called Valtrex.

Genital Warts are similar to Herpes in that they are a virus that remains in your system for life. They are spread in the same way through skin to skin and mucous membrane contact. The warts have to be removed surgically by laser and the bad news is that they may reoccur anyway.

Gonorrhea is a serious bacterial Std that can be spread through unprotected oral-vaginal contact. Symptoms may not show, but vaginal burning, discharge and pelvic pain are common warning signs. The good news is that antibiotics do work, but they must be taken for weeks.

Syphilis is a severe bacterial Std that can also be spread through unprotected oral-vaginal contact, especially if there is a sore present on the mouth or her vagina. Syphilis can be deadly if it isn't cured in the first couple of stages. The first visible sign and stage is the sore at the entrance of the vagina; the second sign is a body rash. Fortunately, Penicillin can cure Syphilis in these early stages. However, the third stage attacks the nervous system and debilitates the heart. Medications have limited success if left untreated.

Crabs and pubic lice are tiny creatures that gravitate towards the pubic hair where they live. They can be spread from one infested person to another. Symptoms include itching, swollen lymph glands and a mild fever.

Hepatitis A is a dangerous virus that can be transmitted by rimming or analingus (licking or penetrating the anal opening with your tongue). Other rimming risks include anal herpes, anal warts, internal parasites and even HIV. Hepatitis A can be prevented by getting a hepatitis A shot. In some cases hepatitis infection can cause muscle ache, fever, loss of appetite, headaches or dizziness.

Hepatitis B can be a life-threatening virus transmitted from sexual contact or contaminated needles. It's found in blood and other body fluids, such as semen, vaginal secretions and the breast of a lactating woman. It's possible to contract Hepatitis B when performing unprotected oral sex, especially when fluids from a carrier enter your body through a cut or sore in your mouth. Symptoms of Hepatitis B are fever, abdominal pain, jaundice and in some cases liver disease. There is no known cure, but it can be prevented with a vaccine.

Hepatitis C is the most deadly of all the hepatitis diseases. It is transmitted exclusively through direct blood contact so the receiver of oral sex must be menstruating, and the person going down on her must have a cut or sore on his mouth. There is no known cure or vaccine for hepatitis C at this time. Symptoms include the same as for A and B, plus dark urine, light stool colors, yellow eyes or skin and tenderness of the liver area.

HIV/AIDS can be fatal when the blood, semen, vaginal secretions or breast milk of an infected person enters another person's bloodstream through a cut, sore or blood vessel. If you perform oral sex on a menstruating partner, you could be at risk. Even if you have recently flossed or brushed your teeth, it's possible that you cut your gums and you could be at risk. HIV doesn't have any immediate warning signs so it's possible to have the virus for years and transmit it to others. The first symptoms of AIDS are weight loss, night sweats, pneumonia and other illnesses related to a low immune system. There is no known cure or vaccine for AIDS, but combinations of medications can slow the virus down.

How to properly put on a male condom

Prepare: Always check your condom for an expiration date, throw it out if it is expired. Also, make sure to store condoms in a cool place, such as a desk drawer, never store a condom in your wallet, hot environments (such as in your car) or if it has been washed or dried by accident. Don't hesitate to get a new condom if you have any doubts.

The penis must be erect in order to put on the condom. Do not attempt to put a condom on if the penis is limp.

Opening: Be careful when opening the package, condoms can rip very easily. Feel free to use your teeth, in a sexy manner, but be careful.
If the man's penis is not circumcised, be sure to pull the foreskin back first.

The condom should be right side out. Make sure to unroll the condom slightly at first in order to check which direction it is unrolling in. Slip it over the head of the penis; moving downward (it should unroll easy). (Hint: try putting the condom on with your mouth, watch your teeth.)

It is important that you hold the top half inch of the condom between your thumb and forefinger when you roll it down. This will leave space for when your man ejaculates.

Roll down the condom as far as it will allow, it should reach the base of the penis.

In the case of anal intercourse (remember: always use a condom during anal intercourse, even if you cannot get pregnant) use a lot of lubricant, the anal region is not naturally lubricated and can tear more easily than the vagina. For intercourse, a water-based lubricant is best. Always apply lubricant after the condom has been put on, a condom could easily slip off of a lubricated penis. Apply lubricant as often as needed, dry condoms break more easily.

For Men: make sure that when you pull out, you continue to hold the condom in place at the base of the penis. If possible, pull out while your penis is still erect. It is imperative that you remove the condom only after you are completely out of your partner's vagina.

Once you have safely removed the condom, throw it away immediately, a condom can be used once, and only once. In the case of anal intercourse, make sure you use an entirely new condom, never switch from vaginal to anal intercourse with the same condom. A man should never ejaculate in the same condom twice, and should also never wear a condom that somebody else has already used.

Also, remember never to use more than one condom at a time. - Doubling Up- only increases the chances of the condom breaking.

Using a female condom

How to properly put on a female condom:

The female condom is a sleeve of polyurethane with a closed end and a larger open end. There is a flexible ring in each end.

Have a condom fashion show

We all need to know about safer sex practices. And, safer sex can be very sexy and fun. For those of you using condoms, experiment with different kinds of condoms and practice putting them on manually and orally.

Condoms:
There are many kinds of condoms including flavored, polyurethane, extra-large, snug fitting, extra-sensitive, and condoms with nubs and stimulators. Here are some examples for you to choose from and experiment with:

Latex: Mentor, Ramses, Durex, Global Protection, Sheik, Pleaser, Kimono, Lifestyles, Crown, Magnum, trojan, Contempo, Paradise

Natural: Fourex, Natural Lamb, Skin Kling

Polyurethane: Avanti, Reality for women (female condom)

New Condoms:
Pleasure Plus Bulbus Head (Gives room inside the condom for the head of the penis to have more friction.)

Custom fit condoms

You can also experiment with dental dams, latex gloves or finger cots.
Safer Sex Activities

- Cuddling and caressing
- Dry kissing
- Undressing
- Phone sex
- Watching or reading erotica
- Cleavage fornication
- Massage
- Mutual Masturbation
- Manual stimulation
- Oral sex with an FDA approved condom or rubber dam
- Sex toys unshared

- Intercourse with a condom and spermicide

Unsafe Sex

- French kissing in the presence of open sores or cuts
- Manual stimulation in the presence of open sores or cuts
- Oral sex without a barrier
- Sharing unclean sex toys
- Sucking the breasts of a lactating woman

- Vaginal or anal intercourse without an FDA approved condom
- Penetration of anything from the anus to the vagina
- Never blow or force air into the vagina because it can cause an embolism that could be fatal, especially if the woman is pregnant.

Birth Control Methods

NuvaRing-99.7%; $30-$35/ monthly. Protects against pregnancy for one month, no pill to take daily, does not require a -fitting- by a clinician, does not require the use of spermicide, nothing to put in place before intercourse. Possible: more regular, shorter periods, less: menstrual flow and cramping, acne, iron deficiency anemia, excess body hair, headaches, depression and vaginal dryness and painful intercourse associated with menopause, reduces the risk of ovarian and endometrial cancers, pelvic inflammatory disease, noncancerous growths of the breasts, ovarian cysts, and osteoporosis (thinning of the bones), fewer occurrences of ectopic pregnancy (in a fallopian tube), ability to become pregnant returns quickly when use is stopped. Increased vaginal discharge, vaginal irritation or infection, cannot use a diaphragm, cap, or shield for a backup method of birth control, rare but serious health risks, including blood clots, heart attack, and stroke (women who are 35 and older and smoke are at a greater risk), change in sex drive and temporary irregular bleeding, weight gain or loss, breast tenderness, nausea (rarely, vomiting, changes in mood, and other discomforts)

Patch- 99.7%;$30-$40/month supply of patches. Protects against pregnancy for one month, no pill to take daily, nothing to put in place before intercourse, Possible: more regular, shorter periods, less: menstrual flow and cramping, acne, iron deficiency anemia, excess body hair, premenstrual symptoms (such as related headaches and depression) and vaginal dryness and painful intercourse associated with menopause, reduces the risk of ovarian and endometrial cancers, pelvic inflammatory disease, noncancerous growths of the breasts, ovarian cysts, and osteoporosis (loss of bone mass), fewer occurrences of ectopic pregnancy (in not in the uterus), ability to become pregnant returns quickly when use is stopped Skin reaction at the site of application, menstrual cramps, may not be as effective for women who weigh more than 198 pounds, rare but serious health risks, including blood clots, heart attack, and stroke (women who are 35 and older and smoke are at a greater risk), other side effects include change in sex drive and temporary irregular bleeding, weight gain or loss, breast tenderness, nausea (rarely, vomiting, changes in mood, and other discomforts).

POPs (Progestin-only Birth Control Pills)- 92-99.7%; $20-$35/ monthly. Can be used by women who cannot take estrogen, nothing has to be put in place before vaginal intercourse, can be used while breastfeeding, ability to become pregnant returns quickly when use is stopped, irregular bleeding patterns, headache, nausea, dizziness, sore breasts, must be taken at the same time of day each day to reduce the risk of pregnancy and irregular bleeding

IUD- 99.2-99.9%; $175-$500/ exam, insertion, and follow-up visit. Nothing to put in place before intercourse, ParaGard® (copper IUD) may be left in place for up to 12 years, Mirena® (hormone IUD) for five years, no pill to take daily, Mirena® may reduce menstrual cramps, ability to become pregnant returns quickly when IUD is removed Increase in cramps and heavier and longer periods (copper IUDs), spotting between periods, increased chance of tubal infection leading to infertility if inserted when a woman has a STI, rarely, wall of uterus is punctured during insertion, rarely, insertion can cause infection, pregnancies, which rarely occur, are more likely to be ectopic (not in uterus)

Depo-Provera- 97-99.7%. $20-$40/visits to clinician. $30-$75/ injection. Can be used by women who cannot take estrogen, nothing has to be put in place before vaginal intercourse, can be used while breastfeeding, effective for 12 weeks, no pill to take daily, helps prevent cancer of the lining of the uterusirregular bleeding, headache, nausea, dizziness, sore breasts, must receive injection every three months, loss of monthly period, change of appetite, weight gain, depression, hair loss, or increased hair on the face or body, nervousness, skin rash or spotty darkening of the skin, change in sex drive, side effects not reversed until medication wears off (up to 12 weeks), causes temporary bone thinning, may cause delay in getting pregnant after shots are stopped, pregnancies, which rarely occur, are more likely to be ectopic (not in the uterus)

Abstinence-100%; Free. No medical or hormonal side effects of any kind. Many people find it difficult to abstain from sex play for long periods of time

Withdrawal- 73-96% (nearly 100% w/condom); Free (or cost of condoms). Can be used when no other method is available. Not effective against Stds, requires great self-control, experience

Sterilization- 99.5-99.9%; $2,000-$6,000/ Tubal sterilization; $350-$1,000/ vasectomy. Permanent protection against pregnancy, no lasting side effects, no effects on sexual pleasure. Risks of minor surgery, regret, usually not reversible, rarely, tubes reopen, allowing pregnancy to occur

The Pill- 92-99.7% $20-$35/monthly. Nothing to put in place before intercourse, more regular, shorter periods, less: menstrual flow, cramping, acne, iron deficiency anemia, excess body hair, headaches, depression and vaginal dryness, and painful intercourse associated with menopause. Reduces the risk of ovarian and endometrial cancers, pelvic inflammatory disease, noncancerous growths of the breasts, ovarian cysts, and osteoporosis (loss of bone mass), fewer occurrences of ectopic pregnancy (not in the uterus), ability to become pregnant returns quickly when use is stopped, can be used to change the timing and frequency of your period rare but serious health risks, including blood clots, heart attack, and stroke (women who are 35 and older and smoke are at a greater risk), change in sex drive, temporary irregular bleeding, weight gain or loss, breast tenderness, nausea (rarely, vomiting, changes in mood, and other discomforts), must be taken daily, persistent side effects may be relieved by having your clinician change your prescription.

Diaphragm- 84-94% $15-$75/ diaphragm
No major health concerns, can be used during breastfeeding. Can be messy, allergies to latex, silicone, or spermicide, should not be used during vaginal bleeding or infection, increased risk of bladder infection, can only be left in place for up to 24 hours

Condom- 85-98% (nearly 100% with withdrawal) $0.50 and up - some family planning centers give them away or charge very little. Easy to buy in drugstores and supermarkets, can be put on or inserted as part of sex play, can help relieve premature ejaculation, helps to protect against Stds and AIDS Latex allergies, loss of sensation, breakage

Female Condom- 79-95% $2.50/per condom Easy to buy in drugstores and supermarkets, can be put on or inserted as part of sex play, erection not necessary to keep condom in place, can be used by people allergic to latex, external ring of condom may stimulate clitoris. May be noisy, may be difficult to insert, may irritate vagina, penis, may slip into vagina during intercourse

Sponge- 68-91% $7.50-$9/package of three sponges. Easy to buy in drugstores and supermarkets, can be put on or inserted as part of sex play, does not interrupt sex play (it can be inserted hours ahead of time) May irritate sex organs, can be messy, may be difficult to remove, cannot be used during vaginal bleeding

Spermicide -71-82% $8/applicator kits of spermicide ($4-$8 refills). Easy to buy in drugstores and supermarkets, can be put on or inserted as part of sex play May irritate sex organs, can be messy

Fertility Awareness- Based Methods (FAMs)-checking temperature daily, checking cervical mucus daily, recording menstrual cycles on calendar, keeping a very accurate record of when your period comes each month, keeping track of your menstrual cycle using a string of beads called CycleBeads 75-99% $5-$8 and up/temperature kits (drugstore).

$13/CycleBeads- Free classes often available in health and church centers No medical or hormonal side effects. Requires expert training before effective use, uncooperative partners, taking risks during - unsafe- days, poor record keeping, illness and lack of sleep affect body temperature and may interfere with the temperature method, changes caused by vaginal infections and douches may interfere with the cervical mucus method, must have regular menstrual cycles that are never shorter than 26 days and never longer than 32 days to use CycleBeads

health information - birth control

If You Choose Fertility Awareness-Based Methods (FAMs)...
... a professional will teach you how to keep track of your menstrual cycle to help you predict -safe- and -unsafe- days. Abstain from intercourse (periodic abstinence) or use condoms, diaphragms, caps, shields, or spermicide during nine or more -unsafe- days

Stds from Unprotected Intercourse
Genital Herpes- Virus; Burning sensation in genitals, low back pain, pain when urinating, flu-like symptoms, small red bumps may appear around genitals, some show no symptoms. Medications prescribed by your doctor, such as ValtrexTM

Gonorrhea-Bacteria Women: strong smelling vaginal discharge, may be thin & watery or thick & yellow/green, irritation or discharge from the anus, abnormal vaginal bleeding, possibly some low abdominal or pelvic tenderness, pain or a burning sensation when passing urine, low abdominal pain sometimes with nausea
Men: white, yellow or green thick discharge from the tip of the penis, inflammation of the testicles & prostate gland, irritation or discharge from the anus, urethral itch & pain or burning sensation when passing urine. Antibiotics (Similar to antibiotics used for Chlamydia)

Chlamydia Bacteria- Women: an unusual vaginal discharge, pain or a burning sensation when passing urine, bleeding between periods, pain

during sex or bleeding after sex, low abdominal pain sometimes with nausea
Men: white/cloudy, watery discharge from the tip of the penis, pain or a burning sensation when passing urine, testicular pain and/or swelling. Antibiotics (those similar to gonorrhea). Such as, Doxycycline

Syphilis- Bacteria; Painless sores or open ulcers may appear on the anus, vagina, penis, or inside the mouth, and occasionally on other parts of the body. During the second stage (roughly three weeks to three months after the first symptoms appear), an infected person may experience flu-like symptoms and possibly hair loss or a rash on the soles and palms -- and in some cases all over the body. There are also latent phases of syphilis infection during which symptoms are absent. Antibiotics. However, can be extremely dangerous if left untreated.

HIV/AIDS- Virus; Most symptoms of AIDS are not caused directly by HIV, but by an infection or other condition brought on by a weakened immune system. These include severe weight loss, fever, headache, night sweats, fatigue, severe diarrhea, shortness of breath, and difficulty swallowing. The symptoms tend to last for weeks or months at a time and do not go away without treatment. In some cases, infections result in death. Doctors can prescribe and array of medications (commonly known as a -cocktail-) to preserve life, however, there is no cure.

HPV (Genital Warts)- Virus; Can cause cervical cancer, visible warts in and around the genitals, may look like miniature cauliflower florets, some show no symptoms. Warts can be removed by a physician, however, they will always return.

SEX THERAPY

In today's prevailing culture, there is a myth that sex is the most incredible experience for the vast majority of people and that is why sex with anyone, anywhere at anytime is always going to be a blissful, orgasmic experience. This myth is continually being sold to us, particularly in the cinema where sex is portrayed as an earth-shattering experience even when the two people having intercourse have only met a few minutes previously. The physical aspect of sex is all that is being portrayed in many of these encounters. The reality of the complex emotional and psychological processes that cause or dampen desire and orgasm are never referred to.

Problems in Sexual Relationships

Much work has been done studying the reasons why many men and women have very unsatisfying sexual relationships. In the 1950s Masters and Johnson carried out many scientific and clinical studies of what causes desire in human beings. Masters and Johnson showed beyond doubt that sexual responses are as susceptible to conditioning as other animal or human behaviours. Sexual functioning in animals and humans is particularly easy to disrupt with punishing external stimuli, and so is especially vulnerable to learned inhibition or distortion.

In the 1970s therapists refined this view of sexual response, based on arousal and orgasm dysfunctions, to consider lack of desire as being a major factor when treating many sexual disorders. Shere Hite (1998) in The Hite Report on Female Sexuality, reported her ground-breaking research into male and female sexuality, based on thousands of detailed questionnaires completed by people in the US. Hite found that many women felt sex was not enjoyable because men usually spent so little time at foreplay and seemed not to understand a woman's need to be fully aroused before intercourse. Many men admitted that early stereotyping of how a real man must perform during sex contributed to much frustration and lack of pleasure in sexual relationships. The feeling that one is emotionally loved and cared about by a partner is also a prerequisite for most people to have a close and fulfilling sexual relationship.

Most people at some time or other feel a lack of satisfaction with or a lack of desire for sex. Our moods, emotions, levels of tiredness and anxiety, and hormone levels may cause this to happen periodically. It is also very difficult for a person who has been conditioned for years to believe that sex is 'bad' or who believes that her body is unacceptable to suddenly feel completely at home expressing her emotions through her sexuality. Sex is the most natural activity in the world, yet because we have been brought up in a very unnatural environment we must accept that problems can frequently occur. Also people may feel under pressure to match cinema standards of sexual performance, believing that 'everyone else has a great time so what's wrong with me'. Many people feel fear, shame, embarrassment, and personal inadequacy when suffering from problems to do with this most personal area of their lives. Due to this fact, the number of people who actually present themselves for treatment is estimated to be vastly lower that the actual incidence of sexual problems.

For those who are continually finding difficulty enjoying the sexual side of a relationship, and especially for those who end up dreading the sexual act but who still want to be sexually active, there are several therapies available to help overcome these problems. The most common sexual difficulties for men are impotence or erectile dysfunction, ejaculatory incompetence or male orgastic dysfunction, and premature ejaculation. For women the most common problems experienced are frigidity or arousal dysfunction, female orgastic dysfunction, and vaginismus or involuntary spasm of the vagina. Lack of desire may occur in both sexes. It has been estimated that about ten per cent of all women never experience an orgasm of any kind.

Psychotherapy and Couples Therapy as Part of Sex Therapy

Specialist therapists offer sex therapy to help couples overcome sexual problems they may be experiencing. For sex therapy to be successful, both partners must commit themselves to attend sessions, to do homework and to try out new techniques for at least an agreed initial period. Individual psychotherapy can be vital to help a person discuss fears, negative conditioning or past traumatic experiences which may be inhibiting desire, arousal or the ability to let go and give oneself permission to have an orgasm. By seeing each person separately the therapist may be able to help clients to talk more openly about their feelings and experiences within the relationship. Their desires and fantasies are also explored. Several sessions with each partner will help the therapist to access the causes of the presenting sexual problems.

Arousal problems are often due to a lack of foreplay or knowledge about what really excites a partner. In couples therapy communication must be opened between partners as to their sexual preferences as this is an important way to help them develop a better understanding of their individual needs. It must be stressed that both people's needs are equally important. Also unless the two people involved really care about each other and want to be together then sexual desire and enjoyment may never really be achieved.

Therapies to Overcome Sexual Problems

Sexual therapy consists of several stages and the couple are encouraged to practise each stage in the privacy of their own homes. Firstly they are requested to massage and caress each other in turn. Then they are asked to kiss and to cuddle, to touch each part of the other's body including the genitals. The next stage is stimulation of the genitals, and of the breasts in women. Self-stimulation may be a helpful learning and sharing process for both partners, followed by then manual masturbation by each partner. If a woman cannot obtain an orgasm using these methods then a finger-tip vibrator can be used. When both people feel comfortable and fully aroused, intercourse can be tried.

Problems occurring at each stage are discussed at the weekly meetings, such as areas of the body that a partner particularly does not like to be touched. Sexual therapy at its most successful leads to a greater deal of open and caring communication, both emotional and physical, between both partners.

SEX ADDICTION FAQ

1. What is sex addiction?

Sex addiction is a way some people medicate their feelings and/or cope with their stresses to the degree that their sexual behavior becomes their major coping mechanism for stresses in their life. The individual often can not stop this sexual behavior for any great length of time by themselves. The sex addict spends a lot of time in the pursuit of his or her sexual behavior/fantasy or they may have a binge of sexual behaviors.

2. Why do people become sexually addicted?

This is different for every sex addict but generally speaking there are biological, psychological, and spiritual reasons. The following is a short explanation of each reason why someone can become a sex addict. The biological addict is someone who has conditioned their body to receive endorphins and enkephlines (brain chemicals) primarily through reinforcing a fantasy state with the ejaculation that provides these chemicals to their brain. Psychologically, the need to medicate or escape physical, emotional or sexual abuse can demand a substance, the early addict finds the sex medicine usually before alcohol or drugs. Spiritually, a person is filling up the God hole in them with their sexual addiction. The addiction is their spirituality, it comforts them, celebrates them and is always available and present. Then there is the sex addict who can be two or even three of the above reasons. This is why a specialist in sex addiction is the best route for recovery with sex addiction.

3. What's the difference between sex addiction and a high sex drive?

I have heard this question on almost every national talk show or radio show I have been on over the years. A person with a high sex drive is satisfied with sex. It's not about a fix for something; when their partner says "NO" it doesn't make them go off the handle thinking their partner is totally rejecting them and have to leave the house or act out in some other way. If you can relate to this the chances are there may be an addiction issue.

4. Can you be addicted to masturbation?

Yes, this is by far the most common sex addiction that I have treated in working with sex addiction. This usually is the first sexual behavior many of us will have on a repeated basis. This is usually where the sexual compulsion starts with sex addicts and this behavior, regardless of other acquired behaviors, usually stays active.

5. What role does pornography play in sex addiction?

Pornography for many sex addicts combined with regular masturbation is the cornerstone for most sex addicts. Many sex addicts have great difficulty getting sober from this combination of behavior. The pornography with fantasy creates an unreal world that the sex addict visits throughout their adolescence and other developmental stages and creates an object relationship that conditions their emotional and sexual self to depend upon these objects and fantasies to meet their emotional and sexual needs hundreds of times before having sex with a real person.

6. Can someone be a sex addict and not be sexual with their spouse or committed relationship?

YES! We call this later stage of sex addiction, sexual anorexia. In this stage of sex addiction, the addict prefers the fantasy world and fantasy sex with themselves or others instead of relational sex with their spouse or partner. The addict/anorexic avoids relational sex and hence this couple has sex infrequently and often at the partners request not the addict/anorexics.

7. What is it like to live with a sex addict from a partner's or wife's perspective?

The partners/wives of sex addicts report many similar feelings about living with the sex addict. The feeling of aloneness is a common experience with partners of sex addicts, the sense that he can't open up and tell you about his "real" self. The confusion of even after you do certain behaviors that this still is not enough and the hopelessness that there isn't enough. Anger for many different unmet needs as a person and as a woman are often common.

8. Can partners get help even if the sex addict doesn't?

Yes, even if the addict stays in denial of their addiction the partner can receive help and support for herself. The feelings of anger, loss, loneliness and many other feelings encountered over the years of living with this addiction will effect a person. These feelings need to be dealt with therapeutically whether they stay married to the addict or not. The addiction was in no way your doing as a partner or wife, the addicts addiction started many years before you even met your addict. This addiction would have grown and damaged anyone they would have related to in any relationship.

9. Is there recovery for sex addiction?

Yes, there is recovery for sex addiction. This recovery takes time and hard work especially in the first year but with guided help the sex addict can experience restoration in their emotional, relational, sexual, financial and even spiritual lives. I have seen marriages made better than they ever were and addicts live much happier lives than they ever thought possible. I have been in successful recovery over eleven years and I know it's available for those who choose to work for and maintain recovery.

10. Is there research on sex addiction available?

There is research being done in the field of sexual addiction. The monitored mail list of Heart to Heart Counseling centers provides weekly research information as well as excerpts from 101 Practical Exercises for sexual addiction recovery as well as Twelve Step discussions.

11. Can women be sex addicted?

Yes! The number of women desiring treatment is growing significantly. The behaviors are the same as their male counterparts including: masturbation, pornography, internet activity, anonymous encounters and affairs. Over twenty recovering female sex addicts contributed in writing She Has a Secret: Understanding Female Sexual Addiction. This book plus the Secret Solutions Workbook, with over 115 helpful techniques for recovery is just for her. If you would like to set up a telephone counseling appointment to start your journey of recovery, call today. There is hope for female sex addicts to recovery.

12. Is there any way to help our children not become sexually addicted?

Yes! Even though many of our adult male clients report that their fathers were sex addicts (porn, affairs, prostitutes etc.) they also report getting little to no proper sexual information to balance their sexual perspective. Good Enough to Wait is the first video of this kind to help your children understand sex and the brain, the long-term affects of pornography, long term sexual satisfaction and a whole lot more. This is the best combination of sex research and spiritual principles to date for youth to watch to give them a proper and currently informed sex talk.

WHY DO MEN GO TO SLEEP AFTER HAVING SEX

One of the most common sexual problems between men and women is that men tend to go to sleep very soon after sex, a time when most women want to cuddle and/or talk. Of course, this is not true in all relationships, but it is true in more relationships than not. In addition to being a frequent complaint, it is also a serious one that can affect not only the sexual relationship but also the relationship as a whole.

It is unfortunate that few men realise the seriousness of this issue, or take steps to address it. For many, going to sleep after sex is completely natural. They do not realise that as they lay snoring away, their partners are laying awake with their emotional needs unfulfilled, often disappointed and angry that their needs and desires for post-sex intimacy have been ignored. These negative emotions are due not only to their needs not being met, but perhaps even more importantly the resulting perception that their male partner is both unaware of and indifferent to their needs. Even in the cases where women have expressed their post-sex intimacy needs, the male partner seldom responds, continuing to fall asleep immediately after sex.

In a long-term relationship, such repeated post-sexual disappointment can easily damage the sexual relationship as well as the relationship more generally. It is an irony that many men seeking to improve their sex lives focus on the physical side (in particular, penis size) and will often spend considerable emotional energy and money on trying to enhance these attributes, when all they need to do to please their partners more is to stay awake a few minutes.

The first step in solving this problem is to understand it. The explanations for why men fall asleep after sex fall into four categories, the first of which is personality related and the remaining three are physical:

- · Indifference. This is the explanation most frequently given by women when asked why men fall asleep after sex. They propose that the man's needs (sexual release) have been met and they are then no longer interested in the woman's needs.

· Oxygen deprivation. Sexual studies have noted that men often hold their breath during sex, especially during climax. A number of articles have concluded that this results in partial oxygen deprivation and attributed the resulting desire to sleep to this.

· Fatigue and/or relaxation. Sex most often occurs late in the day, when men are tired. It also typically occurs in the bedroom, the natural place for sleep. In addition, sex often is relaxing, not least due to the release of sexual tension.

· Hormonal. A variety of brain chemicals and hormones are released during sex; some of which are linked to relaxation and sleep.

The second explanation, while plausible, does not stand up to examination. During sex there is typically a rapid increase in breathing, far greater than required by the physical exertion involved. This elevates blood oxygen and easily compensates for the temporary holding of breath typical at the point of climax. There is little or no oxygen deprivation (this has also been measured in laboratory measurements of volunteers having sex). Furthermore, their are many other activities where men hold their breath (e.g. swimming underwater, pearl divers) or have reduced oxygen levels (e.g. during athletic activities) without feeling an urgent desire for sleep. Although extreme oxygen deprivation (for example, from carbon monoxide poisoning) can induce extreme fatigue and desire to sleep, this is clearly not associated with normal sexual activity.

The third point has more validity. The period between sex and sleep is longer if sexual intercourse is in a place other than the bedroom, if it is earlier in the day, or if it occurs when people are rested rather than tired. It is also true that sleep comes easier and quicker when one is relaxed, so in so far as sex relieves tension, it also inclines one to fall asleep quicker. However, this can only be a partial explanation. Men will often lie awake in bed for long periods before falling asleep, even if they are relatively relaxed. Yet these same men may fall asleep almost immediately after sex. The act of sex, while physical in nature, is not so physically strenuous as to produce exhaustion requiring immediate sleep. Nor is the amount of relation involved sufficient in itself to induce almost immediate sleep. Consequently, while fatigue ard relaxation are factors that play a part, they are only a partial explanation.

The first explanation also provides a partial explanation. Some men are interested primarily in their own desires and once satisfied do not care about those of their sexual partner. However, especially in a long-term relationship, most men want to satisfy their wife/girlfriend and be considered a good sexual partner (even if, as is sometimes the case, it is only so that they can continue to have ready access to sex). It would perhaps be more accurate to say that men have trouble understanding the need for intimacy. For many men, sex is primarily a physical act and once climax is over, sex is completed. They do not see post-sex cuddling and talking as a necessary or even relevant part of sex. Even when this is explained to them by their partners, the concept is often so foreign to their nature that it is difficult for them to understand or respond to it. However, such considerations are only a partial explanation.

The influence of hormones is rather more complex. During sex various brain chemicals and hormones are released, especially at the point of climax. These include norepinephrine, serotonin, oxytocin, vasopressin, and the hormone prolactin. The impact of these various chemicals is only partly understood. However, the hormone prolactin in particular is associated with sleep. Animals injected with the hormone become tired immediately and tend to quickly fall asleep, unless there is a need to stay awake (for example, hunger or fear). The strong link between the release of this hormone and sleep, combined with the release of this hormone during climax, are strong explanations for why men tend to quickly go to sleep after sex. It should also be noted that both the amount of hormone released, and the tendency to go to sleep, are related to the type and strength of orgasm. Research had found that climax from sexual intercourse releases about four times as much of this hormone as climax from masturbation, and that the tendency for men to fall asleep after sexual intercourse climax is much greater than after masturbation climax. A possible hypothesis for further testing is that a more intense climax (better sex), by releasing a greater amount of the hormone prolactin, brings on male sleep quicker. From a woman's perspective, this is perhaps the opposite from what one would want.

In summary, there are various explanations for why men tend to fall asleep shortly after sex. The release of hormones associated with sex (in particular, climax) is a strong explanatory factor. The conditions in which sexual intercourse occurs (end of the day, when fatigued, in bed where one sleeps) along with the release of tension are often contributing factors. In themselves, these factors do not force sleep, but they produce a strong tendency for sleep. Although their female partners may have a strong need to engage in post-sex intimacy, if the male partner is indifferent to or insufficiently aware of this need, the tendency to sleep is not resisted and the man may well go to sleep almost immediately after sex.

COMMUNICATING BETTER SEX

What is sexual communication? In my world, its the ability to reach a level of intimacy that is both fun, exciting, sensual, and helps achieve a better orgasm. Taking the time to understand sexual communication will create the opportunity for a better bond between you and your partner. Even more, some of the traits of the following communication techniques are basic steps to developing a higher level of relatedness with any person. Put them in a different context, and you will have tools to open, create, evolve, and maintain a higher level and more interesting conversation with anyone. Otherwise, consider following for better sex through sexual communication. Give It A Try. It REALLY works!

1. Use Ice Breakers:

Talk about the difficulty of talking, share an article, book movie or other media to open specific subjects. It's highly likely that you both feel nervous about opening up this topic. For example: "Did you see that couple on the news this morning? I was wondering if we could try something like that sometime" (and be OK if your partner doesn't feel comfortable with the request).

2. Use "Active Listening":

Show attention, non-verbally ask for clarification (open-ended and closed ended questions) and paraphrase what you hear until you understand the meaning of your partner's communication. (Paraphrasing means repeating back in your own words what you heard someone say). For example" "So what I'm hearing you say is that it hurts your feelings when I don't kiss you when you walk through the door each night?" Be careful not to turn it into a blaming type of communication. For example "Oh, Great. So what you're saying is that you get pissed just because I don't give you some silly type of attention the moment you come home. Ya know I've had a hard day too! Fine, kiss me then!"

3. Give Feedback on what your partner just said (find the positive parts!)

For example: "I had no idea that I was hurting your feelings and now I can understand how you have been feeling."

4. Empathize with your partner's position, even if you disagree (sense and support the validity of his or her view point or feelings).

5. Use Appropriate Self Disclosure:

Start with small, less vulnerable or anxiety provoking information and be prepared to back off if your partner seems threatened or defensive. The more open you can be, the more open your partner is likely to be, but only IF disclosing is motivated by CARING. Think about how well your partner is able to handle your disclosure and what YOUR intention is (e.g., to bring the two of you closer, help you understand each others needs, or relieve yourself of guilt, or gain power).

6. Compare Notes before and after sex according to your own styles and preferences (e.g. some are more inclined to hint or show rather than tell directly). For example, if you are the non verbal type, then after sex, communicate non verbally, ie, smile, caress his body, cuddle up to him, play with his hair and show him your admiration. Or you can always just tell him what a great time you had and what made it so much fun.

7. Make Requests:

Take responsibility for your own pleasure and make requests, using "I Language" e.g. I would love it if you kissed me there one more time!

8. Give Feedback On you Partners Request:

Each partner has a right to say "no". Appreciate the request, clearly decline (No mixed messages, including non-verbal) and feel OK with your choice. You may possibly offer an alternative.

9. Use Gentle & Constructive Criticism:

- o Do NOT use criticism to blame, hurt, get even or get one-up.

- o Select an appropriate time and place that feels comfortable for both you and the one you are with.

- o Temper with praise - provide compliments and appreciation.

- o Nurture small steps - don't rush for the finish line. Its a process, so appreciate each step along the way.

- o One complaint per discussion - or not at all. Complaints can come off as hurtful or negative and will only set you back to have to work towards gaining trust and respect.

Your presentation is EVERYTHING! How you approach the one you are with will make or break any situation. If you are aggressive and they aren't receptive, you can pretty much end the situation. Know who you are with, which means listening more and talking less will result in a better understanding of what your partner wants, how they feel, and build trust and repoire. Even in long standing relationships, presenting well and building up is always the best approach. Not understanding what transpired during the day, or what is being thought of at the moment will often result in an unfavorable result!

When approaching sex, its often an understanding of the mood and desire of your partner. If you both are showing signs of desire and intimacy, take the time to develop that and stay focused! Know when to talk and when to receive. At this point, everyone is different. One of my favorite movies is "Friends with Benefits" where they finally end up having sex together. They talk about what they want, how they want it, and when they find it, shut up and enjoy it, until they reach their desired orgasm. Now that's hot! This isn't to say that certain positions feel better than others or how sex is happening... but it is to say that if it isn't going the way you want, that you speak up and do so with compassion, understanding, and a desire to get what you want through that perspective: Mutual Satisfaction. Otherwise, if its "all about you", the sex will never be as great as you'd like and certainly not as satisfying.

10. At An Impasse?

Take a break from the topic for awhile and agree to address it at another time, or agree to disagree and accept your partner's view while validating the legitimacy of your own. BE GENEROUS at times, even if it is something that you are not in the mood to do or prefer.

11. Get unbiased support:

If it appears to be a chronic issue, go to counseling together, talk to a respected religious figure, turn to family or friends but do not just ignore the problem, they never just fade away, and the relationship deserves the attention.

It's OK to express your feelings and what you desire, so long as it isn't in the context of a 'put down'. Be open and honest and if you are in a long term relationship that you enjoy, be equally open to your partner's needs. Doing so will allow for practice, practice, practice. And we all know what that means: Practice makes perfect!

Love, Passion, Romance, and Intimacy are the very foundations for a happy and healthy relationship. While other characteristics and intrinsic actions also qualify for a successful relationship, my passion and desire is to bring sex alive and well to every relationship, while addressing the very foundations necessary to do so.

MEN CAN HAVE BETTER SEX

"Honey, it's not a race!" That is what many women will tell their partner during - and especially AFTER - they have sex. And indeed it is not a race. Yet the question is if men can help it if they feel that sex - and especially the actual intercourse - is a physical achievement. Because if you're a man, that is what it feels like.

And it happens for a very simple reason. Men are biologically programmed to do one thing as often and as good as they can: to fertilize as many females, as often as realistically possible. This is because that is what their genetic encoding tells them to do. It is the result of the survival of the species and this is what male mammals do. In fact, that is the prime task of any male species.

While we are not apes or rabbits, and much of this of course is socially unacceptable, that is what evolution has been grinding in for tens of thousands of years. And as much as a modern man doesn't want to procreate non-stop, a large part of this - albeit redundant - genetic encoding is still very much there. And since it took so long to develop, expecting that the individual male will be able to erase it in one lifetime - or even in ten or twenty generations - is totally unrealistic.

Deep down inside - driven by reflexes and not by deliberate reasoning or by choice - men will only want one thing: get in and produce a powerful blast of sperm into the vagina - as far as possible and as much as possible. Again, that is their genetic duty. Their contribution to the survival of the species. For that reason the male orgasm largely feels like an explosion: pressure being built up until it nearly bursts and then he will give everything to blast it out as far as he can. His body will react just like that and will roll all his physical energy and musclepower into one tiny ball of semen and eject it, preferably with "rocket" force. (the reality requires that - although it feels very different - men actually do not exactly "shoot very far". The best of us will manage only a few inches, but then, only half an inch is enough).

Additionally - his genetic reflexes will tell him to do all of this as quickly as possible while holding on to the female with all his strength, so the chances that the female will run and the sperm will not be used for its original design are minimal.

So, genetic encoding tells him: get it in RAPIDLY, get it in DEEP and DUMP THE PAYLOAD, no matter what the cost. The male sex hormones - driven by genetic encoding and cortex reflexes - will tell his body to do exactly that and nothing else. In that sense the human male - like any other male species - is much like a B52 bomber when it comes to sex.

The new gadget: sex for mutual fun

Evolutionary speaking, "sex for fun" is a relatively new gadget that has only been around for the last few thousand years of evolution. Ten minutes or so on the evolutionary clock. "Sex for mutual fun" - again in evolutionary terms - is something BRAND NEW, only discovered a few centuries ago. Hence - regardless how many generations have since passed - it is still something that is very much in the early adapting and learning stages.

Learning is FUN

We told you about the "female side" monkey. Here is one of its cousins: learning is a mutual thing. Men do not just have to learn about the female sexuality. BOTH still very much have to learn about the other.

In fact, learning about sex is largely a very new thing and poorly developed. Something that society in general hasn't even fully adapted. We are still very much supposed to "know" about sex. It is not something you talk about openly and freely (just look at the constant attempts by various governments, religious fanatics and politicians to try and gag those, trying to talk about it freely, for example on the Internet). Which - for example - is why a country like the United States, when it comes to teen mothers, beats the average third world country in the negative sense of the word.

Experimenting, exploring, discovering is NOT WRONG, no matter what politicians or others may tell you. It is how we - the human race - learn. We've learned to identify what types of food are indeed food and which are poisonous by trial and error. Athletes learn by trying to experiment with their body and their abilities. Babies learn by feeling, trying and exploring. Sexuality is no different! And, exploring and learning is FUN. It should be. If it wasn't we would never learn anything!

So, every time she says "Honey, it's not a race!" you aren't doing something wrong. Both of you are! Simply because BLAMING DOESN'T BELONG IN BED.

Communication is the lubricant and the tool that will help both of you (and we'll come to talk about that). Through communication and exploration you'll both find what is fun for both of you. And partners will need to teach each other.

Here is where we are touching on a specific difference between general sex and BDSM. In a BDSM context the power dynamics will be different. As a result, the submissive partner will expect the dominant to set the tone and the submissive will follow. That is usually not very helpful to the situation. BOTH partners - regardless the BDSM dynamics - will have to teach each other and dom/sub dynamics have a tendency to get in the way. Strict role behavior and the natural tendency of the submissive to try and please are likely to form a barrier, leaving one of the partners (partially) unfulfilled and blocking the road to growth. This is where a lot of uncertainties (for dominant partners) and self-blaming (for submissive partners) originates from.

The controlled rat race

So, if it is a rat race, what do you do to avoid it? You may have guessed - for starters you probably can't avoid it. But ...you can learn to control it and turn it into a well organized rat race that is fun for both.

Turning over and going to sleep

"When he's done he turns over and falls asleep." How often have men been confronted with that. And quite frankly, it is not only true, there is also very little he can do about it. The male orgasm is intense, physically intense; and the huge flows of adrenaline, combined with the sudden cut off of the tension and the physical release is what causes him to feel totally exhausted and he needs time to recuperate. Hence, it is NOT WRONG for a man to feel tired and sleepy immediately after an orgasm. It is what his body tells him to do.

Unfortunately, the female orgasm and the male orgasm do not develop at the same pace and as result, by the time the man is done the woman isn't even half way done. And his fatigue - which to her seems to be lack of interest - is her biggest disappointment. As a result, what both of you need to learn is to get your timing right. Which is why introductory play - or foreplay - is so important. Maybe not to him, but most certainly to her.

Unfortunately, during sex the erected penis literally is a loaded barrel, ready to explode any time and the longer it is kept erected, the more likely the orgasm is to come instantly (quite often almost immediately upon penetrating the vagina). And not all men are capable to maintain an erection for a very long time.

A frequently asked question: why is it that nature hasn't taken care of "in sync" orgasms for the male and female? The answer again is in genetics and evolution. If you are a woman, you may want to brace yourself for what is coming.

From the point of reproduction there is no need for a female orgasm. She doesn't need one - at least not as an incentive. She is the passive half of the reproduction process and will be fertilized, orgasm or no orgasm. The man, however, is to be lured into wanting to deposit his seed - hence it should be fun, hence an incentive, hence the orgasm.

That is also why the female orgasm is different from the male. The male orgasm is largely a physical driven one (although fantasy does play an increasing role in the male orgasm) - the female is a mentally (fantasy and emotions/feeling) driven one. For women the concept of sex for fun is much older - simply because the only function of the female orgasm is FUN (in the sense that there is no biogenetical reason for it). So, as far as sex for fun is concerned, the men are several hundreds (maybe thousands) of years behind. They are - sad but very true - evolutionary speaking - still seed-machines. Very efficient machines, but ...still.

That is not entirely true of course. Men too have discovered the sex for fun concept and quite a long time ago. Unfortunately, there are frequent conflicts between what his genetic duties tell his body to do and what his mind wants to do.

So what to do? Well, actually it isn't that difficult. As opposed to widespread urban legends: MEN DO HAVE THE CAPABILITY TO HAVE MULTIPLE ORGASMS. Just not in the same way as their female partners. In other words, it isn't a constant flow (the female "waves of orgasms"). Instead, he needs a bit of time in between before he can charge himself up again. And a simple way to do that is to make sure you eat a bit in between, preferably sugar or chocolate or a banana - anything that will give a quick energy boost. So - have an orgasm, grab a bite to eat (nothing can be more romantic), maybe have a glass of sweet wine and get ready for the next part of the session.

"Honey, was it good for you too?"

On to the the next monkey. Let's face it, your genes don't care if it was good for her or not. Your genes just tell you to dump the load, whether she likes that or not. The problem again is that what your genes tell you to do is not exactly socially acceptable and very likely not even what you want either. But then, genes don't care about social conventions or other motives. They just care about reproduction.

Fact of the matter is that both the male and the female orgasm are VERY SELFISH EXPERIENCES. The orgasm is something for YOU, not for your partner. Neither can "share" the individual orgasm with the other, nor does anyone want to. At best - if you're lucky - you can orgasm simultaniously. But that will still be two individuals, each in their own orgasmic trance.

Hence, the idea is to control the rat race by understanding and a bit of planning. But most of all by NOT WORRYING. Sex does not have to end in an orgasm for both and most certainly not in a simultaneous orgasm. And an orgasm (and especially an ejaculation [cumming]) has long ceased to be an obligation, regardless of what your genes would like you to believe. If either of you "didn't make it", that's perfectly okay. In fact, women especially will often not mind, since the orgasm itself is only partially what sex is about to them. The intimacy, the cuddling, the whatever-else-she-likes will usually be much more important. And, in a BDSM-setting the orgasm will actually be much more of a release valve and not so much the goal of the entire thing.

Four hints for successful sex

1. An orgasm is not a goal, the intimacy is. No orgasm is not a disaster - in fact, the orgasm, yours or hers, is nice to have but entirely unimportant (unless you are really planning to create offspring, in which case HIS ejaculation - which is not the same as an orgasm - IS important).

2. Simultaneous orgasms are PURE LUCK - if it happens it is great, but the chances are 100 to 1 that it won't, so don't bother.

3. The trick is in planning. There are many ways to achieve an orgasm. If you bring HER to an orgasm and masturbate to have your own later, that is perfectly okay, for example. As a man having an orgasm is easy, so the emphasys should be on her - it takes her longer to get there and it takes more effort. So if it is important to you both to have an orgasm during sex, make sure she gets there first. You can either "hop on the train when she's close to the station" or have your own orgasm later.

4. Take the stress out of your lovemaking. Stress is sex and libido killer number one. Stress at work, stress at home, stress in the relationship, financial stress AND stress because you feel your sex has to accomplish something are all very negative influences. Relaxation helps. Make it fun and take your time. Have a shower or even better a bath first (the Japanese have turned bathing into an artform in itself), go romantic, go kinky, go sexy, go exciting, but DO something to take your mind off the daily stress and worries. Creative sex, with regular changes and surprises, also improves your sexlife.

EFFECTIVE WAYS TO BETTER SEX FOR COUPLES

There are proven methods to improve sexual performance and pleasure among couples. However, various couples struggle with different challenges. One couple may be dealing with erectile dysfunction in the male partner, another with lack of sex drive in the female or male partner. Some couples have too much stress in their lives that's not managed properly and this negatively affects their sexual experience and intimacy. For others a lack of creativity is the major cause of disinterest and boredom and has lead to poor sexual performance and desire. The mistake that happens often is when couples use an inappropriate method for treating the problem. You see, all of the conditions listed above are encountered by many couples and each problem requires a unique solution. Additional problems and frustrations occur when a couple uses the wrong method to treat their specific problem, for instance using a drug or other method as the "cure all" for what is lacking in their sexual experience. An example would be someone using a medication or other herbal substance that is intended to treat erectile dysfunction, but that person thinks that the substance will increase sexual desire, which is not the case because that is not how the substance was designed to work.

Erectile Dysfunction

This is also referred to as "impotence" in men. It is the condition in which the male partner has a sex drive (very important), can get an erection (or at least start the process), but is unable to maintain an erection for the intended duration of sex or until an orgasm is reached. This condition is appropriately treated with medications. And you can treat it with natural substances also. The medications used to treat erectile dysfunction belong to a class of drugs called phosphodiesterase inhibitors. Included in this class are the drugs Viagra, Cialis, and Levitra. They are effective in treating impotence because they cause more complete filling of the penis with blood and allows the penis to remain engorged for a longer period of time, usually long enough to reach climax and sometimes even beyond that. Viagra has proven effective in enhancing sexual pleasure in women in a similar way by increasing blood circulation to the vaginal area. Levitra has been proven to help treat erectile dysfunction in men that also suffer one or more other illnesses that compound the problem. Among them are diabetes, high blood pressure, and hyperlipidemia (high cholesterol levels in the blood). There are also natural herbal products that help treat erectile dysfunction without the side effects that may be encountered with these medications.

It is important to consult your primary doctor in determining whether any of the medications are the best option for you, especially if you have a history of heart disease or low blood pressure.

Lack of Sex Drive

This is when there is no desire to participate in sexual activities. There are different causes for this condition. Stress can be a factor. Many medications have decreased sex drive as a side effect. Depression is a cause, especially when it leads to physical inactivity. Even our diets can contribute, directly and indirectly, to lack of sex drive and performance in men and women. It is important to distinguish lack of sex drive from erectile dysfunction, here's why. Let's say a man has no or low sex drive and becomes frustrated because he is unable to become aroused sexually for his partner, yet he believes that Viagra (a treatment for erectile dysfunction) will help solve the problem. He will more than likely become more frustrated because that is not how Viagra works. It was not formulated to stimulate or increase sex drive. With Viagra, Cialis, and Levitra there needs to be sexual arousal which releases certain enzymes or chemicals into the bloodstream that allow the medications to be effective. Without arousal this does not occur. There are some natural ways to increase testosterone levels that have been proven to dramatically increase sex drive. There are even foods that help with this. Exercise is a great way to enhance testosterone levels and sex drive in a safe way, but some forms of exercise are more effective than others.

Stress Anxiety Depression

I put these together because they can be closely related if we don't manage them properly. The mismanagement of stress and anxiety often lead to depression. High stress, anxiety, and depression are major inhibitors of good sexual and general health. It is true that great sex has to do with the right mental stimulation and attitude and nothing negatively impacts the right mind set more than high stress, anxiety, or depression. We manage these conditions by incorporating things that make our lives more balanced. Some ways include; diet and exercise, involving ourselves in more spiritual pursuits, committing more time for the family, or it could be just getting rid of things that make you stressed, anxious, or depressed. Usually effective management involves some of everything. The important thing is that you take action to get them under control. They can be managed effectively by most of us.

Lack of Creativity and Romance

Some couples kill their sex lives when they stop being creative. Even sex, as pleasurable as it is, can become old and even boring if we stop being creative. You see, creativity starts the mental process that sets the stage for great sex. Creativity gets our minds involved in the act. Let's face it, anyone can do it or go through the motions, but to really have great sex involves a bit more from the mind and body together. Remember when you first met your partner and how you felt. The excitement you felt during that time was a motivating force that helped you think up ways to show them how much you cared. And your efforts paid off in a good way, didn't they? I will let you know that by involving the mind in thinking of creative ways to communicate your affection towards your partner can engender the same excitement you felt when you first met. It will make a difference in improving your chances for great sex every time.

HOW TO IMPROVE YOUR SEX LIFE

Many men complain that their wives are no longer as keen in sex as before. This is especially after they have kids and wives usually say they do not have the energy for sex. However, some couples despite their busy lifestyle juggling with careers, children and homes, can still continue to enjoy great sex.

What are their secrets?

(1) Make an effort to improve communication

Communication is how we get to know another person. Make it a habit to chat to one another everyday about how you are feeling. Share your thoughts and ideas, likes and dislikes, feelings and deepest needs with your partner. Ask her what she likes. If you get to know yourself and your partner well through better communication, chances are higher that you will have a much more erotic and explosive relationship.

(2) Do not blindly believe other guys' bragging

When men talk to each other they often exaggerate about their exploits in order to make themselves look better to their peers. This can create distorted pictures of their sex lives for one another. As a result, many guys wonder if they miss anything in their sex life and why they cannot enjoy sex like others.

(3) Accept that sex is never perfect

Do not compare your sex life with porn. What you see in porn is usually far away from reality with perfectly shaped men and women engaging in rousing sex. One of the most destructive myths of porn is that it tries to make guys feel they are too small. Some of the other fictions that porn perpetuates are the idea that women are always ready for sex and that the same moves work on every partner. However, you can use porn to inspire you to greater sexual exploration, but do keep in mind that what you see in porn is not reality.

(4) Focus on the physical sensations

Sex is best when there is no expectation of anything in particular happening. Some guys can get so stressed up because they are worried about performance. To achieve optimum orgasm, simply focus on the pleasurable sensations. Get yourself totally tuned into the moment with her. You can set the tone by teasing her slowly, touching her hands, arms, face, neck and back before going to the more erotic areas. Let her body signals (e.g. change in skin color, her expression, her moaning) guide you to where you should spend more time on any particular erotic spots that she is extra sensitive to your stimulation.

(5) Create a more conducive bedroom atmosphere

If you can do something to transform your bedroom into something new and different, that can make a big difference to your sex life. Lighting some candles or changing the brightness of the room lights to give a more romantic tone is an option worthwhile to consider. Getting a nicer set of sheets and a new bed spread can be of great help. You can give your room more space by removing things like kids' toys, piles of laundry that tends to accumulate in the bedroom. Consider ditching the bedroom TV too or at least trying life without it for a while. Bedroom should be a private place for couples to interact and understand each other better and watching TV is a great distraction to communication.

(6) Arrange time for sex

Some people may feel that this is quite unromantic because in their opinion sex should be something spontaneous. But with modern urban living getting busier and more stressful, not specially setting aside the time for sex may probably result in a gradual decrease frequency in lovemaking.

Rather than giving you a lot of pressure to perform at a particular moment, scheduling can actually make sex more relaxing. You can develop certain sensual rituals, making romantic gestures, sending sexy text messages in anticipation of your encounter. You can give each other a massage or take a shower together. Scheduling lovemaking sessions can also eliminate conflict over differences in sex drives by agreeing beforehand how often both sides should have sex (making some form of compromises).

(7) Make some changes

The changes can involve trying to do something different together to break the routine. This can be making love in different places or trying different lovemaking positions that are mutually enjoyable, or injecting role-playing into your sexual encounter. You can at times do something crazy or extraordinary such as watching horror movies, going for a roller coaster ride, going for trips to unusual places, going for wine-tasting or cuisine-sampling session, enrolling in yoga or dance classes together.

(8) Do not avoid sexual problems

People who have sexual issues often shy away from sexuality because they are afraid to face failure. But these problems need to be addressed head on. Erectile dysfunction gets the most attention but there are other problems too such as premature ejaculation, low libido level, pain during intercourse, vaginal dryness, or difficulty in achieving orgasm caused by medications or medical conditions.

While some sexual problems may need medical attention, others can be solved by trying different intercourse technique. The main thing is not to muddle through your problems and suffer in silence.

Attend therapy with or without your partner. Through therapy, you can work through issues that you have with sex, or bring your partner to talk about how to communicate better so that you can find ways together that overcome the sexual problems. Visit the doctor to talk about your decreasing sex drives so that he/she can come up with certain treatment or therapy or prescribe you alternative medication if the current drugs/pills you take, affect your sex life.

(9) Do not rush

Go slow on sex gives you ample time to build up the sexual tension and make her want you more. Maybe when on the sofa, you can start caressing her and kissing her slowly. Get her in the mood and make her want to take it to the next level herself.

The best sex emerges from whole body sensuality which means you have to switch the focus from reaching the objective to just enjoy the whole process. Leisurely lovemaking benefits both parties. Women get turned on and enjoy sex more, while men have fewer sexual problems and feel more confident about themselves in bed. Many men find that their sexual problems (such as premature ejaculation) subside when they take their own sweet time.

(10) Exercise and proper dieting

If health and fitness are not strong reasons to get you to exercise, how about improving your sex life? Running, walking and swimming can build up your heart endurance. Ex sometimes requires you to hold unusual positions for short period of time and weight training can help to condition your body muscles for longer lasting sex. Doing some stretching exercises after workouts or yoga can help to improve your body flexibility so that you can easily get into any sex positions.

Eat well but be careful not to eat too much especially right before sex. Eating certain food can increase sex drive. Foods that contain Vitamin A, B, C, E as well as Zinc, Selenium, Manganese, Antioxidants, Phytoestrogens are natural sex boosters. Or, you can try foods such as celery, raw oysters and bananas.

(11) Breathing exercises

Take long, quick, deep breaths through your nostrils and then breathe out through your mouth. As you do this, visualize yourself breathing oxygen into your whole body or focusing it on that one area that you want to feel energized. Keep doing this until you feel your body starts to become energized. You can then reach for your bed. During your lovemaking session, continue to breathe in through your nostrils and breathe out through your mouth. Continue this way of breathing and you will feel your body becomes more energized and your endurance increases.

(12) Do not give up

Having a better sex life will need some effort on you and your partner. You should expect setbacks in some of your attempts. Trying something new always involves some risk of failure. The most important thing is to keep trying.

MISTAKES TO AVOID WHEN MAKING LOVE

Everyone wants to have great, hot, steamy sex every time but the reality is that sex in a long term relationship can get a bit stale. Better lovemaking becomes the goal of many couples in this situation who frantically look for new things to try but end up making some bad lovemaking mistakes that actually makes their experience less than what it was before!

In the interests of better love making everywhere here are some of the most common mistakes that lovers tend to making in their quest for better sex.

1. Being Too Scared/Embarrassed To Talk About New Things

This is all too common and really shouldn't be as the person we are making love to should be the person we can communicate with about these things best! Sometimes we may be worried about what they may think however but for the most part your partner will crave new things too so go ahead and ask! It does not need to be crude or kinky but there are thousands of ways to add excitement and passion to your lovemaking that you can explore only if you talk and become comfortable with it!

2. Convincing Them To Have Sex

Oh boy, men mainly make this mistake, but sometime women too! If your lover is not in the mood for sex as they are too tired or distracted then trying to talk them into it is not going to work. Instead you have to raise their arousal levels slowly because when the body becomes sexually interested it releases adrenaline into the system giving energy to make love.

Ladies - If your man seems disinterested in sex but you need some love don't just expect a man to jump at the chance if they really are tired. Instead pay some attention to his manhood by fellatio or by hand.

Men are also visual creatures so wearing something sexy or nothing at all will help! An interesting point is that a man's testosterone levels are highest at 9-10 AM during the day so this is the best time to get him turned on.

Men - Women are very different from us, do not rush in to the obvious sexual areas to turn them on, leave the breasts and crotch alone and concentrate on looking into her eyes, kissing her neck lightly and stroking area near the obvious sexual ones gently. Go slow and when they react positively move to kissing the mouth and so on.

3. Rushing Foreplay To Get To Intercourse

Again many people look at men as the main offenders here but sometimes women do the same and both end up missing out on something amazing. Did you know that lot's of foreplay actually adds to the intensity of an orgasm for both men AND women?

The more you kiss, touch, caress and so forth before the act of intercourse the more aroused we become and more feel good chemicals in our body are produced or build up for the climax. This means that it is ALWAYS a good idea to just slow it down a little and enjoy playing some games with each other and pleasuring them without intercourse for as long as you can before you just have to move on!

4. Getting Sex Toys Or Porn For Your Lovemaking

There is a time and a place for these things but sometimes we tend to rush into these things to soon when we hit a rough patch sexually and it backfires.

Why? Because you do not your lover to end up looking more forward to the plastic toy or watching the porn than actually finding pleasure in each others bodies! Before you include any of these things you need to know how to please your partner in all ways before introducing something else ... use these things as spice and variety not as a central part of your lovemaking.

5. Trying To Climax Your Woman From Just Intercourse

OK Guys and girls listen up. Men, you might feel less of a man if you can not satisfy your girl from intercourse but the reality is that this is not always going to happen and it is not your fault! Some women can not achieve orgasm through intercourse even and those that can sometimes have difficulty depending on a range of factors including the time of the month, hormone levels, mood and so on.

Girls, by the same token do not put pressure on men to make you orgasm from intercourse as there are many other ways to climax if you let your man try some things!

One of the best ways to do this is by mastering the art of cunnilingus (going down on your women). If done right all pressure is off you on the lovemaking because you can make her climax with just your mouth and tongue.

6. Trying For Simultaneous Orgasms

This is seriously overrated, instead of being some mystical moment of combined pleasure where you come as one it ends up being a labor of timing and holding off and stuffing around and when it does happen ... that connection is not actually there.

Instead you should focus completely on satisfying the woman's needs first because women take a lot longer and are harder to climax than a man most of the time. Once you both learn to give totally to the other in lovemaking it becomes even more intense as the connection comes from being able to give such an experience and take it in with all your senses.

That's the secret.

7. Do What Works Best ... Every time

A little sarcasm there ... sorry! While you might understand you need to break out of a routine for better lovemaking some people are afraid to vary too much thinking if it ain't broke why fix it? The reason it 'wear and tear' to take the machine metaphor a step further, while it may not break or fail a boring sex life even if it is still enjoyable can have dire effects on your relationship especially if you also make mistake number one.

Instead be open to change a bit at a time, no need to try new things all the time every time but without spice and variety and excitement sex loses that spark that brings couples together so closely at the beginning of a relationship.

TOP 10 SEX MYTHS

Very few things that happen during sex are a disaster unless you choose to see them that way. When you change the way you look at things, the things you look at will change.

The Journal of Marital and Sexual Therapy recently reported that 1 in 4 of us are unhappy with our sex lives. Problems with sex arise out of a combination of factors: for example lack of confidence, communication difficulties, inexperience and lack of skill, unrealistic expectations, refusal to take responsibility for our own sexual pleasure and

What many people are not aware of is that there are a vast amount of beliefs and opinions about sex that we all have and take with us into every sexual encounter. For the most part, we are not aware of out particular biases and expectations yet these unexamined yet rigid convictions have the potential to ruin any sexual experience.

1. SEXUAL FANTASY IS A BARRIER TO INTIMACY

Many people prevent themselves from having the best sexual experiences that they could have because they believe that fantasy should be restricted to masturbation and should not be an aspect of partner sex. This could not be further from the truth. Choosing whether and when to share a private desire with your partner can be exhilarating. Yet sharing is not the point of fantasy. Fantasy is all about learning what turns you on and exploring your potential to express your sexuality. It is not unusual for women to have trouble reaching orgasm with a partner because of insufficient mental arousal. She probably knows how to orgasm through masturbation but feels too guilty to enter the realm of fantasy when with her partner. The ability to be intimate is enhanced by self-knowledge and confidence and the uninhibited expression and communication of fantasy can bring people closer together.

2. PENETRATION IS THE GOAL OF SEX

Concentrating on the destination rather than the journey is responsible for the burden placed upon men to 'perform' on demand but is only a part of a vastly wider area of sexual possibilities. Penetration is often made the center of sex, yet oral and manual sexual activity is likely to be at least as - and frequently more - satisfying for a woman. When penetration is seen as the 'goal' of sex, then foreplay becomes something that leads to proper sex, rather than being a pleasure in and of itself. When sex is reduced to being a rush towards the man's ejaculation through penetration, then it is no wonder that so many people find sex to be disinteresting and boring. It is more that the definitions of sex in our culture are shallow and trivialize the majesty and mystery that sex can be.

3 MORE SEX MEANS BETTER SEX

Quality versus quantity of sex is likely to be different at varying times. It is unrealistic to expect that sex is always going to be mind-blowing and require a heavy investment of time and effort. Variety is the key. Getting stuck in a predictable routine that both partners play out means that sometimes both quantity and quality suffer. We are surrounded by misinformation about sex. Surveys that tell us how often everybody is having sex (or more realistically, how often people say they are having sex) become methods of establishing a spurious norm of sexual activity that you may try to replicate.

Quality can suffer if you are too intent upon upping the quantity of your sexual experiences. Many people feel under pressure to have a lot of sex but this does not mean that they are going to be a better lover or have better sex. It merely means that they have more sex. Compulsive sexual behaviour can be detrimental to your sense of who you are, what you have to offer, your work, relationships. It can mask low quality sex. Comparing yourself with your perceptions of other people's sex lives is always a destructive mode to get into. The only thing that needs matter to you is your own sexual happiness.

4 I AM JUST NOT A VERY SEXUAL PERSON

Loss of sexual desire is a common concern for many people and it is an issue that has no single cause. When you have persistent thoughts about feeling unworthy, unloved, unwanted and of not deserving of great sex, not attractive enough, you may manage to convince yourself that you just are not very sexual. Everybody has sexual energy and the capacity to express and enjoy a fulfilling sex life. What can happen is that your negative thoughts about yourself mean that you lose touch with the sexual part of yourself and start to feel disconnected from your sexuality. Identifying the internal self-talk that is damaging your sexual expression enables you to begin to re-connect with your sexuality and believe that you are no different to anyone else: you deserve and are entitled to sexual happiness. You will need to change the way you think about yourself or your label will become a self-fulfilling prophecy. If you are looking for evidence to back up a belief, you can always find it. It doesn't make it right or true. It just means you see what you want to see, whatever helps you feel comfortable - even this is only the comfort to be found in what is safe, unchallenging and familiar.

5 BEAUTIFUL PEOPLE HAVE BETTER SEX.

Sex begins in the brain and sexual attraction and energy feed off of factors other than physical appearance. When you make love, you are so much more than your body. This belief feeds off the comparisons you make between yourself and other people. Beautiful people do not have more successful relationships, nor do they have better sex. Sexual fulfillment is about self-acceptance. The way you feel about your body is apparent to other people and can make sex a joy or a disaster. The danger with this belief is that you start to play the game of 'If only'. If only I was thinner, more attractive, more sexually adventurous, then I can have the sex life that I want. When you make your dreams dependent upon some other change, then you reduce the chances that you will find the courage to make any changes at all. There is nothing to be gained by waiting. You need to start taking action to change now.

Your body image and the things you tell yourself about your sexual desirability are important factors that influence your sexual happiness. Whilst valuing your own desirability makes quality sex more achievable, loving your looks alone is no guarantee of a deeper and more solid sense of self-esteem. You can feel desirable but empty of desire. Self-acceptance and learning to love yourself extends beyond appreciating your attractiveness and incorporates an acknowledgment and respect of who you are, what you stand for and what you contribute to the world and other people.

6 THE CHILDREN MUST COME FIRST.

Many couples experience a decrease in their sexual satisfaction after they have had children. Believing that the child's needs should always come first can mean that a total lack of privacy, time, energy and commitment makes sex a distant memory. Having children is a stressful time for every couple and the relationship dynamic will change. Balancing affection and attention between your children and your partner is a challenge that needs to be met head on.

Couples with young children need time alone to focus on each other's needs and desires. They need to listen and respect each other and acknowledge their sexual situation, whatever it is. Being a mother or a father does not mean that you have to give up being yourself. It is important to set boundaries with your young children so that they know and accept that their parents expect privacy sometimes and are not always prepared to rush to fulfill their child's needs on demand.

7. SEX IS NO LAUGHING MATTER

Playing, being silly and laughing are all great ways to deepen intimacy and enhance sexual pleasure. Some people believe that sex must be, can only be, 'romantic' and so attach a great deal of earnestness to the experience. It is possible to learn the benefits of lightening up. When sex cannot incorporate elements of play, it is often an indication of an impoverished emotional connection. Usually, it is not difficult to bring the fun back into sex, even if it feels a little forced at first.

When sex is viewed as about achievement and competition, then lightness and frivolity are likely to be absent. Keep in mind that sex is about whatever works for you and keeping play and foolishness a part of sex can help to prevent sex becoming a stale and predictable.

8. SEX MUST BE A GENEROUS ACT; I WANT TO SATISFY HIS/HER SEXUAL NEEDS

Great sex is both generous and selfish. Most people do get turned on by their partner's arousal and this is fantastic but if you put all your energy into finding out what she/he wants, what about you? Who is giving you what you need? Being prepared to get your own needs met is an indication that you are willing to take care of yourself, rather than relying upon other people to meet your unmet and perhaps unvoiced desires.

Sexual communication is all about clarity, saying what you think and feel. It is also about setting boundaries, discussing what you do not like and both parties must be able to say no and for this to be accepted. If you find yourself having sex because you don't want to hurt the other person's feelings, think about what you are doing. Honour yourself and what you want and share any feelings of ambivalence. This means that intimacy levels can remain high and misunderstandings are not given opportunity to distort your relationship with your partner.

9. PREMATURE EJACULATION IS A SIGN OF A POOR LOVER.

Being unable to control ejaculation is a worry for many men. Most practically, even if you have had an orgasm, don't leave your partner high and dry. Often feelings of shame, failure and anticipating your partner's disappointment mean that his orgasm means the end of sex. It comes back to widening your perception of what sex can be and not being enslaved to ideas about sexuality that are widely circulated in our culture.

In terms of his sexual pleasure, learning how to manage his anxiety about performance and being able to talk to a partner are the most effective ways of building sexual confidence. Some of the informal strategies that are popular in our culture do more harm than good. For example, trying to delay ejaculation by distracting yourself with non-sexual thoughts will do little to enhance your sexual pleasure.
This strategy is more likely to create a feeling of disassociation for him from his own body and the situation that he is in. It may help him to delay ejaculation (although this is debatable) but consciously focusing away from your physical pleasure is unlikely to facilitate peak sexual experiences. Being emotionally present during sex is crucial to sexual awareness and intimacy. It is a far more successful strategy for a man to learn about how to control his ejaculation than to continue to consciously create emotional distance from his partner and the sexual experience.

Tantric sex exploration is a great way to learn the capacity to control male ejaculation as it teaches techniques that enable him to distinguish between orgasm and ejaculation. Contrary to popular belief they are not the same thing!

10. AN ERECTION IS ONE AND THE SAME THING AS SEXUAL AROUSAL

This is a difficult idea for many people to get their heads around. Sexual arousal happens within a context that is emotional, physiological and visual. If you think about the nature of desire and attraction, recognise that it is not always a purely physical response; it involves idiosyncratic and sometimes unpredictable preferences. Sexual desire just does not exist without a sexual context. It is confirmed/reduced by the accompanying emotions and thoughts that you focus on at any time. Men have erections of varying hardness according to how they are thinking and feeling at the time. An erection does not necessarily mean that a man is fully, or even a little, aroused. He may become erect without feeling particularly sexy.

For men who are insecure about maintaining their erection, confusing erection with arousal means that they often rush into sex before they are completely ready. If you habitually move from low arousal into sex, desire may well start to decrease. Part of the reason for this is that many men feel that they may lose an erection if they don't immediately act upon its presence. Having sex in an atmosphere of fear and insecurity is not going to give you the best sexual experiences that you are capable of having.

There are many things that men can do to learn to have more confidence and control over their erections and ejaculatory control instead of ignoring his insecurity and depriving himself of great sexual experiences. Whenever your decisions and actions are motivated by fear and uncertainty, you are selling yourself short in some way or another. Many men are not sure about where their pleasure comes from during sex and experience a lack of understanding about their own bodies that means that they are unaware that their whole body can become aroused. If you are committed to gaining ore control over your ejaculatory response, invest in some of the many interesting and informative guides that enable men to delay ejaculation and become more connected with their sexual potential.

Recognise that the thoughts that you have affect the sex life that you create. Know that you can choose to change the way you think and learn self-acceptance, respect for your sexual self and experience ease, excitement and power in the ways you choose to express yourself sexually.

HOW TO KEEP YOUR SEX LIFE ACTIVE WITH YOUR PARTNER

Wonderful as it is, you won't get to the blissful peak until you remove from your consciousness the phantoms of darkness that have destroyed your respect for sex

Be Sporty

Without sacrificing due reverence for your partner, be sporty and agile, of course, not as though you were an athlete on the field. Sex is not a sport or a demonstration, yet you need your sporty energy and spirit in this ritual of no observances. Eating too much just before sex or taking excessive alcohol tends to make the system dull and without spirit. You must be fully conscious of the infinite joy of the sex periods. You should be able to enjoy every feeling you have in every inch of your body; you should be able to feel the warmth of blood that flows underneath your skin. You can't have this full experience with an over-fed or drunken body. Some people drink to pep up their enthusiasm, they will tell you that, to them, sex is a mere mechanical performance. What a sheer waste of resources.

Be Kids Once Again And Have Fun

Take off those 'I'm Mr. so and so' coats and be yourself. You are young and by every measure youthful. You are a child longing to be nursed, longing to be loved tremendously, and longing to be petted. Inside you are an ever-youthful spirit, a never-dying soul. Remember the games of your youth; bring some of these games into your holy bed just for the two of you, then go on and have fun. In sex, you die a little when you have organism and are re-born. This is the elixir of life and the secret of youthfulness. Develop your game into a holy romance. In one such game, the couple took the game of ludo into their holy bed.

Whoever won demanded his or her partner to take off one item of his or her body clothing. In this way, they won themselves into a romance of perfect joy. Mimic children, talk and talk like children, play like children; be the big children that you are and give yourselves a little pampering - all that pampering that you did not have. Be silly a little - with flashes of 'its nice, isn't it?' rhetoric.

Relax and Tell Your Body To Do So

This is not a race and, if even it looks like one, it has no ending so take your time to have a big start. You may start by doing some yoga exercises or massage each other with a mild good scented oil to stretch and re-stimulate your bodies. That done, sit down quietly and watch your bodies relax. A useful technique for relaxation is to do a few breathing exercises in which you breathe out to the count of 4, hold it to the count of 2, then breathe out to the count of 4. This is known as the 4-2-4 breathing. Relax in-between the sessions; especially when she loses moisture or when the male organ gives up midway. Let go penetration or thrusting at such times and touch the deeper sacred places in you.

Explore eternity together

This is wonderful experience. You will certainly enjoy it when you do it. Let eternity wait while you enjoy infinite eternity. The technique is as follows. Sit on a chair, floor or the tip of your bed. Let your partner sit on you. Wrap your feet around each other if possible. Hold each other tightly and breathe in and out together for some time. Next, take time to discover the fragrance of your breathe and enjoy each others breath. Then, close your eyes gently and float, in the infinite fragrance of each other breath, into eternity. Be in eternity and explore the indefiniteness of eternity; the solemnness of your being,

Make It A Wonder Trip

Another variation of the above guideline, but which comes with incredible results, is to assume a comfortable sitting or squatting position with your partner on you. Wrap your feet around each other as before but this time let his erect penis be inside you - that is, if there is an erection. Let there be no shoving, just sit and feel the gentle waves of energy that surge through your body. Listen to the subtle cries and yearnings of your body, mind and soul; direct all passions into the constant prayer of the heart and spirit. Don't shove, be still but be constantly aware of your bodies and spirit amalgamating into one whole. Thank God for His presence as love and then, if you may, rock gently, feeling the touch of Mother God in her while she feels that of Father

God in you. Be still for brief moments and give thanks. Discover in this, your divinity and infinite capabilities.

Leave The Baggage Of Vampire Passions Behind

Now this is the only instruction, a specific rule that must not be taken lightly. Comply with it at all cost and help make our world a better one.Sex is a creative energy and anything you take into its field is instantly supported by the power of creativity. It must be a lovemaking so that our world may be filled with love. Take to the holy bed your vampires of hate, anger, jealousy, hurt, memory of betrayals and bitterness of all sorts and they will soon become substances of reality in your life.

Of our world is such a state of deterioration, it is because of the lack of awareness of this vital information. You generate evil psyche in your home and affairs if this rules is not observed. In the spiritual world, likes and likes and if the aura of sex (remember it is your creative energy) is evil, it will draw many of its likes to you. Never take the vampire passion to the holy bed. Many a man or woman whom has claimed that by having sex with a particular person their fortunes have reversed are not wrong if the bed has been shared with these vampire passions. The evil thought may have been in you before you went to your partner or might have been in your partner at the time of sexual congress. The creative energy of sex creates what you hold in consciousness at the time of its celebration.

Make time each time for contemplative meditation or solemn prayer before you jump into this new world. Attend to pressing tensions, worries, fears or anxieties that are plaguing the mind.

When You Get There

When you get to the holy bed, take time to do everything; take time to touch and listen to the movement of your touch or the touch of your partner. Smell each other. Make eye contact that says to your partner, 'you're in heaven, I'll like to be your friend,' speaking to each other in tones that seem to say to your partner 'transcend this body and win'. Be ashamed of nothing; sing or laugh if you like doing so. Listen to your senses, to the new music of pleasure it sings; feel and discover your sense.

Direct your partner by eye contact, body movement or gentle sighs and words, to wherever your body yearns for a touch those sports gently or in the manner you like most. Leave the past and the future and be present in your body. Let the world wait, the gods are at worship.Leave anxieties behind; do not be anxious for an erection or intercourse and entertain no expectation for orgasm.

Let things just flow and feel the magic, the electricity that runs through you, uniting you. There are infinitely new things to discover in your partner each time - find one each time. You are in a sacred moment, respect what you are doing and do not be an actor. There is no one to impress but you yourself. Be present with your partner and not in your fantasies. Be attentive to the moment of your partner's orgasm and enjoy it. After orgasm, do not leave each other while the spiritual electricity of creativity surrounds you; hold each other in love. Lie in a comfortable position so that you can hold each other longer, strengthening the bond of your union.

Make regular time for this wonder of the universe. All your efforts are to reach out to your being, and this is the moment of the deepest communion with your being. Feel the gratitude of your heart and spirit with each lovemaking. Above all, know that you are creating whatever is in your consciousness in the hours of lovemaking.

Let Sex Be God's Blessing To You

When sex I recognized for what it is - a holy and divine creative power of God in you - it will instantly become a blessing in your life. Sex express love more than anything else you can imagine; it gives you the desire to go on in life for much longer, even towards immortality. Sex, divinely employed, makes you better and better, nurtures and strengthens you. Sex is a journey into the infinite. It gives you the liberation that comes only from the mystic union with all life through the union with your partner. Sex is the overwhelming celebration of your divinity. Respect it now and always and allow its energy to flow out from you to heal the world and enrich it. What can break a marriage when its sex life is holy and perfected?

How Often?

As advised, there must be no rules. What is important is that you make time to enjoy the glory of God in your sexuality. Make sure at such times that you are not disturbed and that you have complete privacy. If necessary, unplug the telephone and settle the children. Usually such available times are in the night. If it should be in the night, make sure that you are not overly tired.

A gentle look at nature reveals that a woman releases just one egg in a month. In one ejaculation, however, a man releases an average of fifty million spermatozoa, enough to populate a whole nation. Nature does not create such a waste; it releases so many sperms because the journey to the sacred egg is an arduous task and many fail on the way. However, not all sex acts are for the purpose of procreation. Sex is for spiritual procreation as well. Attainment of the spirits of peace, love, health and holy visions could also be the purpose of the sex act.

A woman may freely reach orgasm as many times possible, but for the man, it is a waste to ejaculate more than four times in one month. The ideal situation is to ejaculate once a month. Remember that every spermatozoa released has spiritual capability to form a whole human being. These are inner disciples and they love your dearly. Pray before each sex act, and during ejaculation or orgasm, feed your disciples (the released sperms or the orgasm energies) with purpose.

Never waste you sex energy; convert them to other creative energies. A prayer like 'May the love of me flow forth to bless this planet with peace, 'said with a concentrated thought is very effective. Your target may be any person or condition other than the planet Earth.

Keep Up The Fire in the Passion

Never quench the spirit; life is romance. The egg in the woman is sought after millions spermatozoa. That is what the woman must always be. She must present herself such that she is always sough after. She must be seductively mysterious like the egg she carries; vary herself such that her man does not quite know what to expect in the next lovemaking. Sometimes she must present herself commonly and at other times expensively.

Too much of explicit exposure destroys the mystery. Even though your man has seen your nakedness several times, hide yourself sometimes as though he has never seen it before. For the man, know that your woman love surprises; find where she may be taken off guard and woo her over and over. Find from what sense your woman receives communication and woo her often from that sense organ. For example, a woman receives communication from sense of hearing will love you say 'I love you' than buy her flowers. If possible, take trip away from home; the change of venue can spice up the passion.